THE PERSON IN PSYCHOLOGY
A Series Edited by Theodore R. Sarbin

On Emotions, Needs,
and
Our Archaic Brain

On Emotions, Needs, and Our Archaic Brain

Robert Beverley Malmo

Allan Memorial Institute
McGill University

HOLT, RINEHART AND WINSTON, INC.
New York   Chicago   San Francisco   Atlanta
Dallas   Montreal   Toronto   London   Sydney

Library of Congress Cataloging in Publication Data

Malmo, Robert B.
  On emotions, needs, and our archaic brain.

  (The person in psychology series)
  Includes bibliographies.
    1. Neuropsychology.   2. Psychology, Physiological.   3. Electromyography.
I. Title. [DNLM: 1. Anxiety.   2. Neurophysiology.   3. Psychophysiology.
WL102 M256e 1975]
QP360.M34   612'.8   74–6356

ISBN: 0–03–078455–7

To Helen

FOREWORD

CONTEMPORARY CLASSROOM TEACHERS of psychology place a high value on diversity when they select reading materials for their students. University and college teachers like to choose from among full coverage textbooks, anthologies, journal articles, and small books that focus on specific topics. While there is an abundance of textbooks, anthologies, and journal articles, the supply of small topical books is limited. To meet the need for small textbooks that deal with important aspects of the study of persons, the Person in Psychology series was established.

The series is devoted to in-depth reporting of relevant subjects which are frequently included in college courses identified as: "Personality," "Socialization," "The Individual and Society," "Stress and Adaptation," "Abnormal Psychology," "Personality and Culture," "Clinical Psychology," and "Personality and Adjustment."

In selecting topics for the series, the editor has tried to steer a middle course between overly broad areas of study such as "Motivation" or "Cognition" and highly specialized themes such as "Child-Rearing Patterns in Three Island Communities" or "Bargaining Behavior among Ghetto Youth." "Cognition," on the one hand, is too broad a topic for a small book; on the other hand, "Bargaining Behavior among Ghetto Youth," while timely, is too specific for most undergraduate courses. The titles of the books published thus far indicate the not-too-broad, not-too-narrow concept of the series. They are: *Beliefs and Values* (by Karl E. Scheibe), *Aggression and Altruism* (by Harry Kaufmann), *The Concept of Self* (by Kenneth A. Gergen), *Sex and Identity* (B. G. Rosenberg and B. Sutton-Smith), and *How to Do Psychotherapy and How to Evaluate It* (John M. Gottman and Sandra R. Leiblum).

The present volume is a welcome addition to the series. *On Emotions, Needs, and Our Archaic Brain* is an engaging introduction to neuropsychology. A wise admixture of clinical case studies and research reports introduces the student to an important segment of modern psychology.

For a series concerned with the person, Professor Malmo's approach to the neuropsychological components of human action is especially appropriate. Other volumes in this series emphasize the person as actor, as doer. Now Professor Malmo adds a unique discourse on the contribution of the brain to the study of action. He presents and supports the thesis that the primary function of the brain is motoric behavior, that is, action. His clinical reports and systematic studies abundantly illustrate how human action is constrained as a result of brain function.

Unlike many neuropsychology writings that engulf the student in neuroanatomy and physiology, this book takes into account the premise that the reader is interested in human conduct. Professor Malmo wisely avoids overwhelming the student with technical jargon. He defines and illustrates those terms that are necessary to the exposition. He takes the student through the clinic and the laboratory and, step by step, shares his knowledge about the brain, as it functions, in the service (or disservice) of the person.

University of California   Theodore R. Sarbin
Santa Cruz, California   *General Editor*

PREFACE

THIS BOOK IS BASED, to a large extent, on my research over a thirty-year period at the Allan Memorial Institute, McGill University. A substantial amount of this work was done with the cooperation of patients at the Institute, but much of it was also done with nonpatient volunteers. During the latter years I have also been engaged in neuropsychological research with animals.

My research has profited greatly from association with fellow McGill scientists (especially D. O. Hebb and the group of psychologists whom he attracted to McGill) and with D. J. Bélanger and his colleagues at the University of Montreal.

Basically, the entire book is brain-oriented (that is, neuropsychological). From the beginning of my graduate studies in psychology I have had a deep interest in brain function. At Yale I was fortunate to begin my doctorate training with C. F. Jacobsen in R. M. Yerkes' laboratory, to learn neuroanatomy from H. S. Burr, and to be associated with J. F. Fulton and the outstanding group of neurophysiologists that he had drawn to Yale (including J. G. Dusser de Barenne, H. E. Hoff, M. A. Kennard, W. C. McCulloch, and T. C. Ruch).

In Yerkes' Yale laboratory, from Yerkes himself and from H. W. Nissen and W. F. Grether, I gained a deep appreciation of the extraordinary value of research with animals in working toward an understanding of people. I profited greatly from the fine examples of discipline in experimentation and theory construction set by C. L. Hull, C. I. Hovland, the Marquises, N. E. Miller, the Miles, O. H. Mowrer, and the Sears at Yale, and by the McGeochs, A. W. Melton, and H. N. Peters at the University of Missouri. From F. McKinney's example at Missouri I observed how it was possible to apply sound experimental methodology to clinical problems. Although I did not realize it at the time, this example was to be most useful to me later on (in my own experimental-clinical research at McGill).

During World War II, I left my neuropsychological research to take internship training in clinical psychology at the Norwich, Connecticut, State Hospital. Following my internship I was appointed psychophysiologist at the National Institute of Health (then still in the singular) in Bethesda, Maryland.

When I came to McGill in 1945, I set up a psychophysiological laboratory and commenced a series of studies in which cooperation from patients and the residents and staff at the Institute was invaluable. In many of these studies C. Shagass was co-worker. H. H. Jasper's generous advice (especially during this early period) is gratefully acknowledged.

Early in our psychophysiological research we came to appreciate the extraordinary value of electromyographic (EMG) recording. J. F. Davis (our biomedical engineering colleague) and our technical staff (R. Quilter, W. Mundl, and D. Ross) contributed mightily to the development of our EMG (and other) apparatus. J. F. Davis' *Manual of Surface Electromyography* has been of great help to EMG workers; and some of his other important research contributions are listed with the references in this book. In working with EMGs one can hardly fail to see the importance of the motor system for psychological functions.

The book begins with the story of Anne, a patient of S. Barza's. This collaboration with Barza is representative of a number of useful collaborations with psychiatrists to whom I owe much; others were W. Kohlmeyer and H. F. Müller. The work on hypnosis also described in Chapter I was done with T. J. Boag (who was also a collaborator in other research). The hypnotist was B. B. Raginsky. J. Cumberland was the psychiatrist who collaborated with us in recording EMGs from the hallucinating patient. D. E. Cameron introduced me to the important problem of chronic anxiety. Chapter II gives an account of our psychophysiological research on anxiety.

F. H. Davis was an important contributor to our research on tension headaches, described in Chapter III. Chapter III and Chapter IV present combined data from work with Institute patients and nonpatients. Much of the work from our laboratory was done in collaboration with graduate students, to whom I owe much for intellectual stimulation as well as for their research contributions, which they published independently in most instances.

The skilled assistance in data taking and data reduction from a large number of laboratory assistants was indispensable in this research. Outstanding contributions were made by Janet Gardner, Ruth Hubel, and Irene Kohlmeyer.

In writing this book, my greatest debt by far is to my wife, Helen, who assisted with every aspect of preparing the manuscript and who helped work through many difficulties. The manuscript was read in its entirety by Alex Schwartzman, and an early draft was read by Ruth Calman. Parts of the manuscript were read and criticized by Vern Boxell, Edmund Jacobson, Charles Osgood, and Alfred Smith. To these and other colleagues, including some of my graduate students, and particularly to Theodore R. Sarbin, editor of this series, I am indebted for criticisms and suggestions. I was most fortunate in having the careful and critical assistance of Catherine Morency, Pamela Sidney, and Susan Weber in the preparation of this manuscript.

While this book serves to bring together certain experimental findings from our laboratory, its purposes are much broader than this. The book is designed to teach undergraduates something about psychophysiology and neuropsychology. Technical jargon is avoided and essential technical terms are defined throughout the book. A considerable amount of relevant research from other laboratories is presented.

Working with problems such as chronic anxiety, tension headaches, and cardiovascular distress made us aware of some apparent limitations inherent in the ways our brains function. *Archaic brain* in the title refers to these and other limitations, some of which are discussed at length in the book. Archaic brain is *defined* in the concluding chapter.

Montreal, Quebec   R.B.M.
August 1974

CONTENTS

On Emotions, Needs, and Our Archaic Brain

I

Emotions and Muscle Tension: The Story of Anne

ANNE, AN ATTRACTIVE YOUNG WOMAN, resented many things that her mother did. In particular, she blamed her mother for keeping her ignorant about sexual matters. After many angry disputes with her mother, Anne left home and stayed with a friend. However, she returned and began to complain of faintness, dizziness, and buzzing in the ears. Then one morning she awoke to find herself totally deaf.

Anne was nineteen when she came to our psychiatric clinic. She was referred by a doctor who had examined her thoroughly but could find no physical basis for her deafness. After six weeks of psychotherapy, Anne remained totally deaf. However, she learned lipreading, which enabled her to engage in a conversation. Her psychiatrist (who put her lipreading ability to a critical test) thought her deafness had roots in her wish to be free from her mother's nagging voice.

Regarding her older sister Kay as her mother's favorite, Anne had always felt rejected by her mother. Lately Anne's resentment of this favoritism had intensified. She believed that Kay and her mother talked about her. When Anne entered the room she had noticed that their conversation stopped suddenly. Occasionally she overheard them in a nearby room talking disparagingly about her. Her father was not unkind but she felt deprived because he was so unaffectionate.

When the patient became ill and subsequently lost her hearing, the family were deeply worried and they suddenly became supportive. Anne came to the Institute Day Hospital every morning and returned home every night, being accompanied both ways by some member of her family.

One day Anne's therapist injected her with sodium amytal during interview. In part, this was a test for malingering. Hysterics[1] often lose their symptoms under sodium amytal (a barbiturate, one of the hypnotic drugs), whereas malingerers generally go on pretending, under the drug. Anne's behavior was typical of the hysteric. She was able to hear again until the effects of the drug wore off; and later she had amnesia for this temporary recovery of her hearing.

From the recorded interview it was evident that she tried hard to recall the sodium amytal interview. In her words: "I've been trying to think about it, but I can't reach it. I don't know what happened." At least part of this forgetting was undoubtedly due to unconscious (that is, unreportable) repression of a relatively unacceptable memory. However, the forgetting could have been a manifestation of state-dependent forgetting, which is the failure to recall in a nondrugged state what happened to the (conscious) person during the time he or she was under the influence of a drug. This effect was first discovered by Overton (1964), and it has since been confirmed many times.

There was general agreement that Anne was a genuine case of hysterical deafness, now very rarely seen. Despite therapy, the symptoms looked more and more irreversible; therapeutic innovation seemed to be called for. At this point the therapist suggested that we might learn something by measuring Anne's muscle reaction to sudden loud sound, although startling noises in everyday life situations had no overt effect. For instance, the therapist tried to produce a startle response by clapping his hands behind Anne's head, but this failed to elicit any visible reaction. By measuring her muscle reaction, we hoped to find out something about the nature of her deafness.

Measurement of muscle action potentials has been used by relatively few persons engaged in psychological research. A recording of muscle potential is called an electromyogram or EMG. When a muscle contracts, an electrical impulse is generated along the muscle fiber. This electrical impulse spreads from the muscle to the skin. The total amount of voltage at the skin varies with the number of muscle fibers that contract simultaneously. The more muscles that contract, the greater the voltage.

---

[1] Sudden sensory loss (such as of hearing or vision) in a person who believes in the organic character of the deafness or blindness is regarded as a hysterical symptom, and the person is referred to as a hysteric. The differences between malingerers and hysterics are not absolute. However, the distinction between the two is generally regarded as a valid one.

To obtain an EMG, two electrodes are placed on the skin over the muscle (see Figure 1.1). The electrodes pick up the minute voltages (measured in microvolts, or millionths of a volt), which are amplified and then recorded on paper as a tracing.

Anne came to our electrophysiological suite where we put electrodes over muscles in her head, neck, and arms. During the experiment she lay on a bed and wore earphones through which we transmitted a loud sound (see Figure 1.1B).

The first loud tone startled Anne. The EMG recording revealed a sudden, strong contraction of muscles in her neck (see Figure 1.2). After the startle reaction, her head began to tremble and the trembling spread to the rest of her body. A few seconds later she began to weep. Her therapist entered the room to reassure her. When he asked if she had heard the sound, Anne replied that she had heard nothing but had felt pain "as if something hit me on the head." Later she added, "It felt as if the top of my head was going to blow off."

The second loud sound, one minute later, produced no muscle response at all, nor did any subsequent sounds. However, after Anne stopped weeping, she continued to blink frequently. It is possible that the blinking may have been a residual reaction to the loud sound.

In the first test, Anne's symptom defense was broken. Penetration of the barrier was probably due to the novel situation and the intense sound. But—and this is the most remarkable thing—in the sixty seconds that elapsed between the first sound and the second, the functional block against sound was somehow strengthened so that it was now completely effective against even a very loud tone.

The auditory test given to Anne is one that we have given to many persons in our laboratory. From our experience we can say that Anne's failure to show an EMG response to the second loud tone was unique, except for two hypnotized persons whose hypnotic inductions and EMG responses in the auditory test will be described presently.

From the therapeutic point of view, we failed to produce a lasting change in Anne. So we decided to try classical conditioning. A survey of the literature showed that conditioning had been successful in treating conversion hysteria in a number of cases. And, as early as 1912, V. M. Bechterev, a Russian psychiatrist, claimed successful treatment of hysterical deafness with conditioning techniques (see Malmo, Davis, & Barza, 1952).

Anne's therapist suggested to her that the conditioning procedure would help her regain her hearing. (By this time, Anne had become quite proficient in lipreading.) He added that in his opinion she should not expect her hearing to come back during the procedure but that she would be able to hear again the following morning.

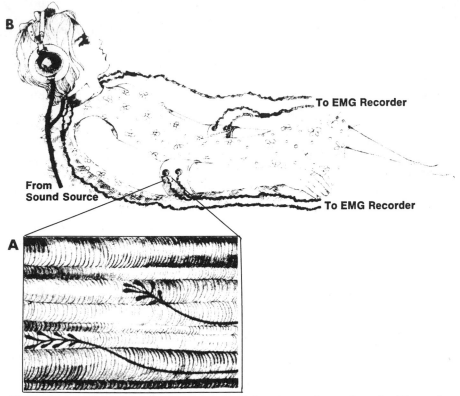

Figure 1.1A *Measuring muscle-action potentials.*   A muscle consists of millions of tiny fibers enclosed in connective tissue. The muscle is activated by a motor nerve which breaks up into fibers that connect, usually in a one-to-one relation, with single muscle fibers in what is called the end-plate region. When an electrical nerve impulse arrives at the end-plate region, it triggers release of acetylcholine, a chemical transmitter, which depolarizes the muscle fiber. This produces a self-propagating electrical impulse that sweeps over the entire muscle fiber, activating the physicochemical mechanism which causes the fiber to contract. The acetylcholine is rapidly destroyed by the enzyme cholinesterase, and contraction of the fiber will cease unless impulses continue to come in over the motor nerve. Each time an electrical impulse passes along a muscle fiber, some of the electrical activity spreads from muscle to skin. The more muscle fibers that contract simultaneously, the greater is the total voltage at the skin. Electrodes are placed on the skin over the muscle, and the signals they pick up are. amplified and recorded as electromyograms or EMGs. For a more detailed account of muscular contraction see Milner (1970). (From Malmo, 1970. Art by Joyce Fitzgerald. Reprinted from *Psychology Today* Magazine, March 1970. Copyright © Ziff-Davis Publishing.)

Figure 1.1B *Recording electromyograms (EMGs).*   The strength of a muscular contraction correlates with the amplitude (vertical movement) in an EMG tracing. The greater the muscular activity, the greater is the amplitude of the tracing. An integrating device developed in our laboratory by J. F. Davis reduces the amount of data produced in EMG studies by converting raw tracings into time-averaged units. The EMG can be used to measure muscle contraction that produces movement (isotonic contraction) or muscle tension without movement (isometric contraction). The EMG measurements are particularly valuable because they can reveal muscle responses that produce no visible movement. (From Malmo, 1970. Art by Joyce Fitzgerald. Reprinted from *Psychology Today* Magazine, March 1970. Copyright © Ziff-Davis Publishing.)

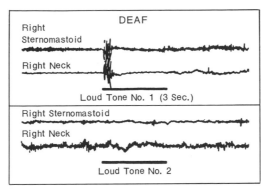

Figure 1.2 *Breaking the barrier.* Anne's first exposure to a sudden loud sound broke through her deafness barrier and startled her. The top EMG tracings show a sudden, strong contraction of her muscles. In a second trial one minute later, the same loud sound produced no effect, nor did any subsequent sounds. During the one minute between the first and second sound, some kind of neural change occurred that completely blocked out EMG reaction to the second sound. (After Malmo, Davis, & Barza, Total hysterical deafness: An experimental case study. *Journal of Personality, 21,* 188–204. Copyright 1952 by the Duke University Press.)

Bear in mind that restoration of hearing was the therapist's main object. Whenever he thought strong suggestion might work, as in this case, he tried it. Scientific procedures were carefully observed in general, but the patient's interests always came first.

During the sessions, Anne sat in a chair and placed one forefinger on a silvered button. She was told to raise her finger each time she felt a shock and then to put it on the button again. A sound was presented one-half second before the shock. Muscle potentials were recorded from both muscles for flexing and extending the forearm.

For the first 149 trials, the tone always preceded a shock. On the next trial, the shock was omitted. There was no detectable finger movement but the EMG recordings showed bursts of muscle potentials (see Figure 1.3A). Both the extensor muscle (used to lift the finger) and the flexor muscle (antagonistic to withdrawal of the finger) showed activity. This conditioned response to the sound continued to appear in most of the subsequent trials when the shock was omitted. It could also be observed after the tone (and before the shock) on many trials when the shock was not omitted.

Our sensitive EMG apparatus was able to detect a muscular conditioned response that otherwise would have escaped observation. The fact that there was muscular activity is significant. It means that the inhibition underlying hysterical deafness was not complete. Some of the neural impulses produced by the sound got through to the motor system. But the influence on the motor system was weak and Anne was not aware of it. Clearly, a powerful inhibitory mechanism was at work.

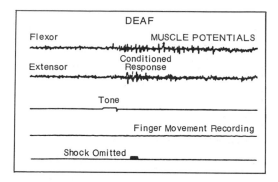

Figure 1.3A *Conditioned response.* For the first 149 trials a sound always preceded a finger shock. On the next trial the shock was omitted. Although Anne's finger did not move, the EMG showed that her finger muscles contracted. Thus, even though Anne could not consciously hear, she exhibited a conditioned response to sound. (After Malmo, Davis, & Barza, Total hysterical deafness: An experimental case study. *Journal of Personality, 21,* 188–204. Copyright 1952 by the Duke University Press.)

After the session, Anne smilingly asserted that she could not hear. Her therapist repeated his suggestion that her hearing would return the next morning. He made certain that Anne read his lips correctly, by asking her to repeat what he had said.

The next morning as Anne was crossing a busy street, a driver who had narrowly avoided hitting her honked his horn and shouted at her. Anne's hearing suddenly returned. It seems that the therapist's suggestion, in combination with the conditioning and with other factors unknown,

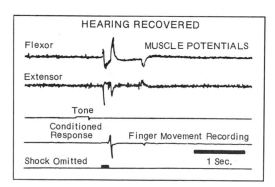

Figure 1.3B *Hearing recovered.* After Anne recovered her hearing, the conditioning session was repeated. Sound and shock were paired for the first 148 trials. Then shock was omitted. Anne's conditioned response consisted of lifting her finger when she heard sound. The recorded muscle potentials were due to the finger movement. Readers interested in other technical points may consult the original source for detailed explanation. (After Malmo, Davis, & Barza, Total hysterical deafness: An experimental case study. *Journal of Personality,* 21, 188–204. Copyright 1952 by the Duke University Press.)

somehow produced the breakthrough that restored her hearing, which remained intact thereafter.

Two days after Anne recovered her hearing, we repeated the conditioning session with her. This time, when the shock was omitted after the tone, the conditioned response consisted of actual withdrawal of the finger from the button (see Figure 1.3B). The bursts of muscle tension that had been the conditioned responses when Anne was deaf did not recur. The muscle potentials recorded on the EMG were due to the lifting of Anne's finger (conditioned response) when she heard the tone.

HYPNOTIC DEAFNESS

Anne's hysterical deafness is an example of a psychoneurotic disorder that somehow makes available a source of central inhibition not normally available. Similar inhibitory mechanisms seem to be involved in hypnotic states. We found two women in whom hypnotic deafness could be induced (Malmo, Boag, & Raginsky, 1954). After one exposure to the startle sound, one woman could suppress muscle reaction to the same extent that Anne did. The other woman showed no reaction even to the first sound. But in the normal waking state, try as they might, they could not avoid showing a strong EMG reaction to the first several sounds even though they had been exposed to it repeatedly while they were hypnotized.

For comparison with these cases of functional deafness we tested a woman who had been totally deaf following surgery at the age of five. As expected, this woman showed not the slightest EMG reaction to the first loud sound. This control was useful in demonstrating that Anne's reaction to the first sound was a breaking through of the deafness barrier and not merely a reaction to some other form of stimulation, such as pressure.[2]

In closing this chapter, we should pay particular attention to the usefulness of electromyography in the study of Anne. Though deafness is a sensory loss, the key role played by the skeletal muscles should be underscored. As will become increasingly clear as we proceed through this book, the surprisingly dominant role of the motor system seems more significant for psychology than has been recognized in recent years.

[2] For further details concerning these investigations, the reader may consult the following references: Malmo (1970) and Malmo, Davis, and Barza (1952). The present scientific status of hypnosis and the trance state is discussed cogently by Hilgard (1973). I agree with Hilgard that there is solid *behavioral* evidence supporting the view that hypnotic induction procedures produce a (trance) state, which is different from the normal waking state, in the same *sense* that the sleeping state is different; although the trance state is clearly quite different from sleep. Also with Hilgard, I respect the views of skeptics who believe that more evidence is required in order to clinch the point. Clearly more research is needed in this difficult area.

SUMMARY

A rare case of deafness was described. During the period of deafness, various medical tests showed that Anne's auditory apparatus was intact. Other tests indicated, however, that she clearly resembled deaf persons in her failures to respond normally to sound. In short, Anne's case was a classic example of the hysteric.

In the study and treatment of this case, electromyography was extraordinarily useful. It may seem paradoxical that deafness, which is sensory in character, should be illuminated by electromyography, which records from the motor system. However, as this book proceeds, the paradoxical appearance of this observation should diminish because one of the main guiding principles involves the unique importance of the motor system for all kinds of behavior, including perception.

In referring to the absence of a normal startle response to loud sound in hysterical and hypnotic deafness, the concept of inhibition was introduced. A powerful inhibitory mechanism appeared to be available to these functionally deaf persons in the startle test, and to Anne in the auditory conditioning series. Precisely how this inhibitory mechanism works in cases like these will probably remain a mystery for some time to come. However, the neurophysiological mediation of inhibition will be explained in Chapter VII in connection with the problem of chronic anxiety, which is the topic of the next chapter.

REFERENCES

Hilgard, E. R. The domain of hypnosis: With some comments on alternative paradigms. *American Psychologist*, 1973, *28*, 972–982.

Malmo, R. B. Emotions and muscle tension: The story of Anne. *Psychology Today*, 1970, *3*, 64–83.

Malmo, R. B., Boag, T. J., & Raginsky, B. B. Electromyographic study of hypnotic deafness. *Journal of Clinical and Experimental Hypnosis*, 1954, *2*, 305–317.

Malmo, R. B., Davis, J. F., & Barza, S. Total hysterical deafness: An experimental case study. *Journal of Personality*, 1952, *21*, 188–204.

Milner, P. M. *Physiological psychology*. New York: Holt, Rinehart and Winston, 1970.

Overton, D. A. State-dependent or "dissociated" learning produced with pentobarbital. *Journal of Comparative and Physiological Psychology*, 1964, *57*, 3–12.

II

Chronic Anxiety

THE PATIENT complains of *persistent* feelings of "tension" or "strain," of frequent irritability, unremitting worry, restlessness, inability to concentrate, and feelings of panic in everyday life situations. The severity of these feelings has been increasing over a period of some weeks. Insomnia is more and more a problem. From time to time the patient is overwhelmed by fright (without apparent cause). The patient finds his work efficiency seriously impaired, and he reaches the point where he believes that he is seriously ill, or even about to die. He goes to the doctor, who says: "I can find nothing wrong with you."

This is a description of someone with *chronic anxiety* (or anxiety neurosis), a disorder which affects about 5 percent of the people on our continent. It is important to bear in mind that this disorder is a *chronic* condition, as distinguished from *acute* states of fear, whether or not the object of the fear is perceived. The term *anxiety*, as it is used in this book, will invariably refer to an enduring state (usually of some months' duration).

Recently, attention was again focused on the cumulative effects of the stresses of war, in Vietnam. Reports indicate that during the Tet offensive, people in Saigon began showing the deleterious effects of prolonged tension. With the onset of indiscriminate bombing, burning, and rocketing, symptoms that were commonplace in World War II (combat fatigue, flying fatigue, war weariness) apparently became widespread. In World War II it was found that if at the first symptoms of developing anxiety—lack of appetite, insomnia, high heart rate, increasing irritability

—the soldiers were withdrawn from active combat and rested for a period of time, many could go back and fight again. However, when the symptoms were not heeded and the soldiers were subjected to continuous pressure and danger, eventually they would reach the breaking point and rest treatment would not bring relief. Instead a chronic anxiety condition would develop.

The same kind of condition is found in civilian populations far removed from anything resembling battle conditions. The stresses in everyday life, when they are prolonged, appear to produce similar effects, although the stresses are sometimes hard to identify. The distinguishing feature of chronic anxiety is that the person afflicted with it reacts to ordinary life situations as though they were emergencies.

The symptoms of chronic anxiety include disturbed breathing, increased heart rate and blood pressure, and increased tension of the skeletal muscles.

While feelings of tension are vague and not amenable to direct measurement, there is nothing vague about the measurement of changes in muscle tension. However, very little research has been conducted on the degree of muscle tension in psychiatric disorders. Is the level of muscle tension greater than normal in all types of psychiatric patients? Do the muscular responses of psychiatric patients to "emotional stress" differ from those of "normal" persons? To answer these and other questions, we carried out some experiments in our laboratory with patients showing symptoms of chronic anxiety and with a group of normal persons.

It is worth noting that these experiments were conducted before the advent of tranquilizing drugs. We were able, therefore, to study the relatively unaltered condition of chronic anxiety. Such studies would be difficult to arrange today because physicians routinely prescribe tranquilizers for "anxiety."

In previous experiments, we found that EMG and other physiological measurements taken while a person was at rest could not be used to differentiate between normal persons and patients with chronic anxiety. So we decided to measure the startle response in order to compare *anxiety patients* with controls. In selecting patients, we adopted clinical criteria of anxiety, which conformed to the diagnostic practice in our Institute, and which was as simple and straightforward as possible. Accordingly, we defined "anxiety" as a tensional state of such severity that work efficiency was impaired and medical advice was sought, and which was characterized by one or more of the following complaints: persistent feelings of "tension" or "strain," irritability, unremitting "worry," restlessness, inability to concentrate, feelings of panic in everyday life situations. As Sarbin (1968) has pointed out, "anxiety" is a potentially troublesome term. To be explicit, we chose anxiety patients on the basis of the criteria listed above, and then we proceeded to compare the physiological reactions of these patients with those of control subjects, under controlled conditions of stimulation.

During the experiment, the person lay on a bed. Muscle potentials were recorded from the extensor muscles of the right forearm. The startle response was induced by a sudden loud sound through earphones.

The anxiety patients exhibited slightly greater muscle tension than the normal persons at the beginning of the experiment, but the difference was not statistically significant. With the onset of the sudden sound, the average rise in muscle tension was nearly identical for the two groups during the reflex period (2/10 second) of the startle reaction. Then there was a difference: "normal" persons returned to prestimulation levels within ½ second after the sound, while the muscle tension of "anxiety patients" continued to rise, and their residual high-level muscle tension extended over the entire three-second period of auditory stimulation (see Figure 2.1A).

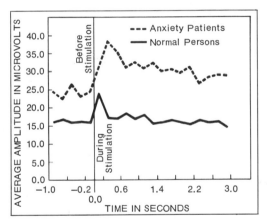

Figure 2.1A *Prolonged tension reaction in anxiety.*   When startled by sudden sound, both groups show a comparable rise in muscle tension the first 2/10 second. In normal persons muscle tension drops quickly; but in anxiety patients tension continues to rise and remains high over the entire period of auditory stimulation. This indicates that in persons with chronic anxiety the regulatory mechanism that brings muscle tension back to a relaxed state is not functioning normally. (After Malmo, Shagass, & Davis, *Science*, Vol. 112, pp. 325–328, 22 September 1950.)

The results show that anxiety patients are not different from normal persons in their primary startle reaction: it is in the recovery phase that the difference occurs (see Figure 2.1B). This reminds one of G. L. Freeman's (1948) concept of "residual load," which covers undischarged excitation effects left in the system after stimulation. According to Freeman, a low residual load refers to physiological recovery (deactivation) in a situation where the individual responds fully and appropriately to an environmental change and then relaxes. Individuals who are repeatedly unable to relax, when relaxation is appropriate, carry a high residual load, which is evident in physiological recordings.

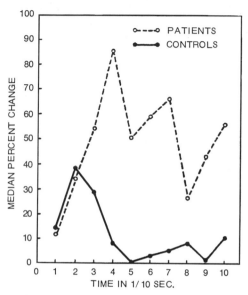

Figure 2.1B *Percent change in EMG response.* During the first second of stimulation, change in response shows that the difference between patients and controls is in the after-reaction. Curves show median percent change in EMG. (Zero percent represents level preceding stimulus.) Note nearly identical response (change) of patients and controls during the first 2/10 second. But note that from 2/10 to 3/10 second the controls' curve falls while the patients' curve continues to rise. Patients' curve reaches a peak at a time when controls' curve is down almost to prestimulus level. (From Malmo, Shagass, & Davis, *Science*, Vol. 112, pp. 325–328, 22 September 1950.)

I believe these observations provide important clues about the fundamental nature of chronic anxiety. Overactivation of the skeletal muscles is clearly involved. With this point in mind, it is of considerable interest to note that some biochemical research with chronic anxiety patients also suggests a link between chronic anxiety and activity of the skeletal muscles. Four investigations in four countries have shown that, under controlled exercise conditions, blood lactate is significantly higher in chronic anxiety patients than in normal individuals. When muscle fibers contract, they convert large quantities of glycogen (glucose sugar in its storage form) to lactic acid, most of which diffuses into the blood.

Interestingly enough, Pitts (1969) has found, in a series of well-controlled studies with anxiety patients, that he could induce some of their symptoms (for example, heart pounding, breathing difficulties, apprehensive feelings) by injecting them with lactate.

We are all aware that there are certain physiological changes, such as increased heart rate, blood pressure, and breathing rate, which accompany muscular exertion. The physiological mechanisms involved in these activities will be discussed in Chapter IV. We turn now to the results of some further research with anxiety patients, in which various physiological measurements, in addition to EMGs, were taken under controlled conditions. Because the reactions of anxiety patients to mildly painful stimulations were particularly interesting, we will commence with these experiments.

ANXIETY PATIENTS AND PAIN

In experiments designed to extend our observations of physiological deviations in anxiety, we recorded from anxiety patients (selected according to the criteria previously stated) in a situation where painful stimulations were administered. For comparison we also took recordings from normal control subjects.

We used a modified Hardy-Wolff thermal-pain apparatus, in which light from a 500-watt lamp is focused on a person's forehead, which is blackened with India ink in order to increase heat absorption. The person tested sat forward with his chin in a support (see Figure 2.2). He was told to expect a sensation of warmth on his forehead that might suddenly swell into a stab of pain. He was instructed to press a button with his right forefinger when he thought the heat on his forehead was about to become painful.

Twelve stimuli of brief duration were given at intervals of exactly 1½ minutes. This meant that the stimulations were carried out over a period of 18 minutes. Physiological recording was continuous throughout this entire period. We were just as much interested in the physiological recordings between stimuli as we were in the immediate (phasic) reactions to the stimuli themselves.

Figure 2.3 shows samples from two typical records, one from an anxiety patient and the other from a matched normal control. The physiological tracings illustrate some of the differences between groups that proved to be statistically reliable after analyzing the data from all persons tested.

Anxiety patients signaled pain more frequently than normals. Normals never withdrew their heads from the chin rest; but most of the anxiety patients did so, at least once. Breathing irregularities during stimulation were much more common in the anxiety-patient group (see Figure 2.5 for an illustration of this difference).

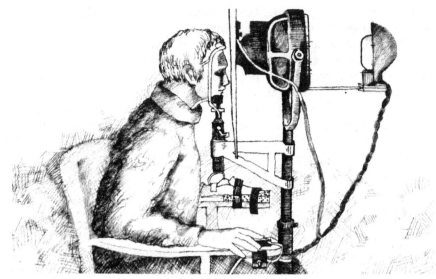

Figure 2.2 *Pain stimulation apparatus.*   During stimulation, light from a 500-watt bulb is focused on the person's blackened forehead. The right forefinger rests on a button with crystal pickup which records pressure on the button (to signal pain) and also finger movements ("tremors") throughout the 18-minute test period. Electrodes placed on the neck for muscle-potential recording, and the pneumograph around the chest for recording breathing are not shown. Left hand is shown strapped down for galvanic skin recording (GSR). The person's chin rests in a support and his forehead is placed against two metal stops at the top of the frame. Persons taking the test are asked not to remove their heads during stimulation. (From Malmo, 1970) Art by Joyce Fitzgerald. Reprinted from *Psychology Today* Magazine, March 1970. Copyright © Ziff-Davis Publishing.)

The foregoing are examples of discrete (that is, *phasic*) reactions to the stimuli. A brief physiological reaction to a stimulus is called *phasic*, as previously noted. The distinction between phasic and tonic physiological measures is an important one to keep in mind; this point will be detailed later. Now let us note some differences of the *tonic* variety—physiological measures based on recordings over the entire 18-minute period.

Bursts of finger movement (tremors) and bursts of neck-muscle potentials were far more frequent over the 18-minute period for anxiety patients than for normals. In a subsequent study, tonic levels of arm-muscle potentials and blood pressure were recorded and found to be significantly higher in anxiety patients than in normals.

To some extent, the results support the view that anticipation of pain is especially arousing for patients with pathological anxiety. However, they are also overactivated physiologically in situations where pain is not involved.

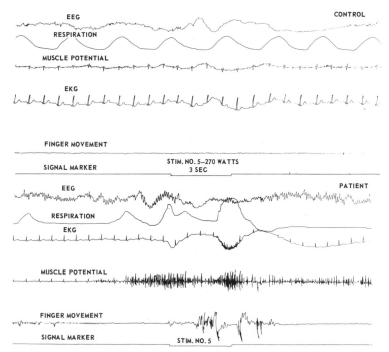

Figure 2.3 *Comparison of anxiety patient and normal control.* Patient: Thirty-three-year-old male chemist with chronic anxiety neurosis. Control: Thirty-three-year-old male physician. High-anxiety patients signal pain more frequently at lower heat intensities than normals (270 watts was lowest intensity used, 500 watts the highest). High-anxiety patients also show more bursts of muscle potentials and more "tremors," between stimuli, than do normals. (From Malmo & Shagass, Physiologic studies of reaction to stress in anxiety and early schizophrenia. *Psychosomatic Medicine*, 1949, *11*, 9–24.)

PHYSIOLOGICAL RECORDINGS FROM ANXIETY PATIENTS IN SITUATIONS NOT INVOLVING PAIN

Finger-movement irregularities (tremors) were much more frequent in an anxiety patient group, compared with normals, in our Rapid Discrimination Test. The person being tested was seated in a darkened room and asked to view a screen on which were projected six circles, like those shown in Figure 2.4. The task was to choose the largest circle and to call out its number before the next set of six circles appeared on the screen. Finger movements (tremors) were recorded from the left forefinger which simply rested on the recording button all during the test. There were 20 sets of circles, presented three times.

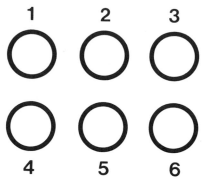

Figure 2.4 *One of the sets of circles used in our Rapid Discrimination Test.* Task is to view circles projected on a screen and to call out number corresponding to largest circle before the next set of six circles appears on the screen. Finger movements ("tremors") are recorded continuously from the left forefinger. High-anxiety patients had significantly more "tremors" than normals. (From Malmo, Shagass, Bélanger, & Smith, Motor control in psychiatric patients under experimental stress. *Journal of Abnormal and Social Psychology*, 1951, *46*, 539–547. Copyright 1951 by the American Psychological Association, and reproduced by permission.)

Arm-muscle tension (EMGs), blood pressure, and heart-rate levels were also abnormally elevated during this test. Differences between anxiety patients and controls were confined to the physiological measures. The patients performed as well on the test as the normals.

Figure 2.5 presents blood-pressure data from another test situation, again with no pain involved. The task was to trace around the outlines of a circle while viewing the hand in a mirror. The person must learn to revise his habitual way of drawing in order to adjust to the reversals in perception caused by the mirror. This mirror reversal makes the task difficult.

Blood-pressure level in psychoneurotics[1] (who were mainly anxiety patients) climbed higher and higher all through the test. Even the normals' blood pressure increased as they listened to the instructions and as they commenced the task; but then their blood pressure stayed at the same level. Here we have evidence of the anxiety patient's physiological reaction rising higher when the normal's reaction is being checked. This is the same kind of difference we noted in the startle test. Here the change is *tonic* (over minutes); there it was *phasic* (within a few seconds).

Figure 2.5 shows that it is not just any group of psychiatric patients

[1] According to the classification of the American Psychiatric Association, psychoneurosis is a behavior disorder without clearly defined structural change in the brain. Patients with chronic anxiety represent a large subgroup; other manifestations of psychoneurosis are reactive depressions, phobias, and obsessive-compulsive behavior. Strict boundaries between behavior disorders do not exist, and we must be careful to avoid false generalizations.

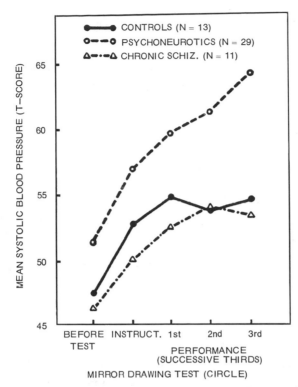

Figure 2.5 *Blood-pressure changes during Mirror Drawing Test.* Majority of psychoneurotic patients in group were high-anxiety. Blood pressure in this group continues to rise while that in controls is leveling off. On this measure, the blood-pressure changes for a group of chronic schizophrenic patients appear normal. Blood-pressure readings were converted into *T* scores, which help to prevent factors of age and sex from influencing results. (From Malmo & Shagass, Studies of blood pressure in psychiatric patients under stress. *Psychosomatic Medicine*, 1952, *14*, 82–93. See p. 85 of this article for explanation of *T* scores.)

that will respond with unchecked rise in blood pressure. The "high-anxiety" psychoneurotics are obviously a group apart.

Psychophysiologists agree on the conclusion that regulatory mechanisms are defective in anxiety. Lader (1969) in his comprehensive and critical review clearly establishes this point. It is a general finding that, under a variety of conditions, high-anxiety patients continue to be over-activated physiologically, when normals have returned to baseline. The reader who is interested in pursuing this topic further may consult Lader's chapter for references to the original articles.

The evidence for this conclusion has been drawn from observations of both phasic and tonic physiological changes. This distinction is of such fundamental importance in psychophysiology that it deserves special comment.

DISTINCTION BETWEEN PHASIC AND TONIC PHYSIOLOGICAL CHANGES

Phasic reactions are brief reactions, lasting over only a few heart beats. A *tonic* heart-rate change, on the other hand, is a shift in *level* persisting over hundreds of successive heart beats.

Tonic Heart-Rate Change in Anne

When deaf, Anne's resting heart rate during the three minutes prior to her startle test was at the level of 98 beats per minute, compared with 74 beats per minute prior to the test after recovery of hearing. We may assume that the latter was close to her normal resting heart rate. The rise in heart rate to a *level* of 98 beats per minute before the first test was a *tonic* change. Despite our efforts to reassure her, it is obvious from her high heart rate that Anne was apprehensive about the test. This is hardly surprising considering the special significance of a hearing test for Anne at that time.

Effects of Reassurance before Testing

In our physiological studies of patients with anxiety, we were usually more successful with presession reassurance than we were with Anne. As a result, we were often able to bring patients' physiological levels down nearly to normal values before the test. Under these circumstances, it is easy to understand why we generally found our most reliable differences between patients and normals during the test rather than in the pretest period. This, of course, does not necessarily mean that our patients were more "reactive" physiologically than patients in studies by others who might report reliable differences between patients and controls in the pretest period, and not much greater differences thereafter. It could mean merely that our initial period of pretest preparation and reassurance was longer, and therefore more effective.

It is plain that a physiological function that is already highly activated will generally react less to further stimulation than one that is less activated. It is absurd to call a person whose muscle tension is already extremely high, "low in physiological reactivity" simply because some stimulus does not cause much further rise in muscle tension. It is a well-established principle in psychophysiology that any phasic reaction must be judged in relation to the tonic level prevailing at the time.

This seems to be the sense of Lader's (1969) caution against using the term "reactivity" too loosely in psychophysiological studies of "anxiety." The point is that chronic, excessive physiological change, phasic *or* tonic, is characteristic of anxiety patients. The one which happens to predominate will depend on the precise conditions, before, during, and after testing.

SUMMARY

From the classical research of Walter B. Cannon, we know that Nature has provided us with physiological mechanisms designed for short-term intense muscular exertion in emergencies. These mechanisms provide activation and support of the skeletal muscles, which will be the subject of the next chapter.

Activation of strong contractions is largely a function of the sympathetic nervous system, which will be discussed in Chapter IV. In mobilizing the resources of the body for intense muscular effort, one of the things that the sympathetic nervous system does is to provide an increased blood supply to the muscles. This means an increased heart rate and blood pressure, and a shifting of blood from the outside of the body (in the skin) internally to the muscles. These and other conditions assist the muscles in breaking down glucose and extracting *energy* from it for vigorous action.

In this physiological mobilization for action, the adrenal gland, located above the kidney (see Figure 4.1D) plays an important role. The inner part of this gland (adrenal medulla) secretes a hormone, *adrenalin*, into the blood stream. Adrenalin (or epinephrine) is the *chemical transmitter* for the sympathetic nervous system, which will be considered in Chapter IV. For the present purpose, it will be sufficient to know that adrenalin in the blood stream speeds up the mobilization of muscular energy. In the process, there is an excess of lactate in the blood. Normally (that is, after a brief period of energy mobilization), the lactate is resynthesized into glucose in the liver.

From our infrahuman ancestors, we have evidently inherited these mechanisms, which Nature designed for short-term emergencies of primordial fighting and fleeing. It is also evident that when these mechanisms are activated too frequently, there are undesirable consequences.

In battle anxiety we see the effects of a prolonged period in which the serviceman faces one emergency after another. This means that the man is called on repeatedly for extraordinary action. Not only in meeting each emergency, but also in preparing for new ones (and even in reliving old ones), the classic emergency physiology of Cannon is applicable.[2] In fact, the physiological mechanisms described by Cannon carry one

---

[2] For excellent detailed descriptions of these experiences in airmen, see Grinker & Spiegel (1945).

through many stressful episodes with little or no residual effects (as G. L. Freeman, 1948, explains). But prolonged exposure to situations of this kind eventually produces the chronic condition of anxiety. Some individuals reach this chronic condition sooner (and with apparently less stress) than others. This may be chiefly a matter of constitutional pre-disposition. Yet even men regarded as stable by psychiatrists fall victim to anxiety, if their exposures to these demanding situations are prolonged enough (see Grinker & Spiegel, 1945, p. 85).[3] These consequences may be viewed as one line of evidence that our brains are archaic. The archaic feature seems to involve a set-point that remains elevated after it should have returned to a normal level. This principle (of a "sticky" set-point) will be discussed in Chapter VII.

Finally, we again call attention to the outstanding importance of the motor system (that is, the brain mechanisms controlling the muscles). In the next chapter this theme will be elaborated.

REFERENCES

Freeman, G. L. *The energetics of human behavior*. Ithaca: Cornell University Press, 1948.

Grinker, R. R., & Spiegel, J. P. *Men under stress*. Philadelphia: Blakiston, 1945.

Lader, M. H. Psychophysiological aspects of anxiety. In M. H. Lader (Ed.), *Studies of anxiety*. Ashford, Kent: Headley Brothers, 1969. Pp. 53–61. (*British Journal of Psychiatry, Special Publication No. 3*).

Malmo, R. B. Emotions and muscle tension: The story of Anne. *Psychology Today*, 1970, *3*, 64–83.

Malmo, R. B., & Shagass, C. Physiologic studies of reaction to stress in anxiety and early schizophrenia. *Psychosomatic Medicine*, 1949, *11*, 9–24.

Malmo, R. B., & Shagass, C. Studies of blood pressure in psychiatric patients under stress. *Psychosomatic Medicine*, 1952, *14*, 82–93.

Malmo, R. B., Shagass, C., Bélanger, D. J., & Smith, A. A. Motor control in psychiatric patients under experimental stress. *Journal of Abnormal and Social Psychology*, 1951, *46*, 539–547.

Malmo, R. B., Shagass, C., & Davis, J. F. A method for the investigation of somatic response mechanisms in psychoneurosis. *Science*, 1950, *112*, 325–328.

---

[3] The conditions that eventually produce chronic anxiety are obviously complex. From reports of psychiatric observers in the front lines, one of the most important factors is the exceedingly intense effort which the battle situations demand. Another important factor, in most individuals apparently, is the necessity to perform acts (such as killing people) that run counter to all previous training, and (hopefully) to natural inclinations of human beings. For example, an airman must dive his plane to destroy and kill. This requires tremendous concentration and effort. At the same time, for most airmen, it is a revolting thing to do. This prolonged high-level con-centrated action performed in the presence of aversion to the act appears to have serious physiological consequences.

Pitts, F. N. The biochemistry of anxiety. *Scientific American*, 1969, *220*(2), 69–75.

Sarbin, T. R. Ontology recapitulates philology: The mythic nature of anxiety. *American Psychologist*, 1968, *23*, 411–418.

III

On Tension Headaches, Motor Functions, and the Brain

DISCOMFORTS RELATED TO OVERACTIVE MUSCULAR CONTRACTIONS

TENSION HEADACHES and other discomforts that are related to overactive muscular contractions have been studied in our laboratory by means of electromyography. These studies, some of which are described below, throw light on physiological mechanisms underlying tension headaches and related pains. They have a further usefulness in suggesting one of the archaic (and troublesome) features of the human brain.

Overactivity of Muscles Specifically Associated with Tension Symptoms in the Absence of the Symptoms during EMG Recordings

Case 1. Complaint of Cramping Feelings in Muscles of the Left Thigh
The patient, a forty-two-year-old woman, came to our psychiatric clinic complaining of difficulty in falling asleep, irritability, and of being sensitive to noise. Her most distressing symptom apparently was severe spasms of the left thigh.

The patient had suffered periodically from discomfort (cramping feelings) in her left thigh for some thirteen years. She had been getting these cramping feelings in bed at night, which made sleep difficult. Noises, which irritated her very much at any time, seemed to be especially unpleasant for her at night, and they seemed to trigger off the cramping sensation in her left thigh.

It may be significant that the patient recalled some unpleasant childhood memories about her father coming home late at night, drunk, and beating her mother. She lay in bed, fearful of what would happen when her father came home, and was unable to sleep. She listened for the sounds of her father coming in, and for the sounds of his attack on her mother.

In the laboratory we asked the patient to point to the center of the area on the left thigh where the pain appeared. We placed a pair of electrodes where she pointed. This was on the lateral surface of the vastus externus muscle, about six inches directly above, and in line with the lateral bony prominence of the knee region (that is, the lateral condyle of the femur). As a control (to test the specificity of the muscle reaction) we placed a pair of EMG electrodes on the opposite side of the body, on the right thigh. They were placed so that they corresponded exactly to those on the left. Other electrodes were placed on other regions of the body.

EMG recordings were made while the patient performed in a tracking test. The procedure will be described from the point of view of an observer, in the control room of our duplex laboratory suite, viewing the patient through a one-way vision glass.

Figure 3.1 shows a picture of a person taking the test. She turns a knob, which controls the movement of a needle in an electrical meter. Her task is to make the needle that she controls follow (or "track") the movements of the other (apparatus controlled) needle, up and down the meter scale. Wires attached to eight muscle groups over the patient's body are led to a plugboard, which sends cables through conduits in the wall into the instrument room where the investigators are watching the eight oscillograph pens writing on moving paper. We note that the EMG amplitudes are approximately the same from one channel to the next. The patient is working quietly at her task and there is no sign of rising tension in any muscle.

Now, however, the conditions under which she is working are changed. By means of a tape recorder, disagreeably loud sounds are sent through a loudspeaker in the patient's room. With the presentation of these distracting loud noises there is no observable change in the patient's behavior. (She has heard these sounds before so that they do not startle her.) She carries on tracking and were it not for the oscillograph record, we would conclude that the sounds were having no effect on the patient. But watching the oscillograph record, we see a clear change in one of the channels,

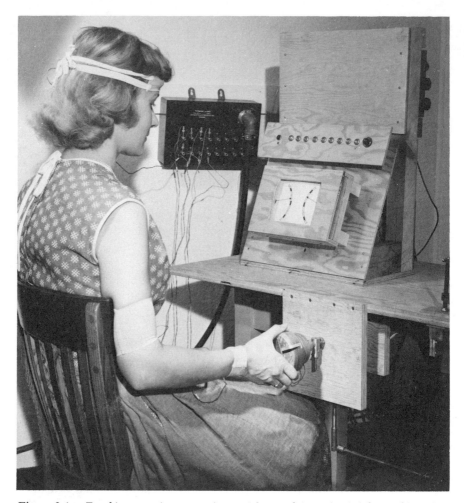

Figure 3.1. *Tracking test given to patients with complaints of painful muscle tension.* EMGs are recorded from muscles causing discomfort, and from other muscles. By rotating the knob the person controls the movement of one of the needles in the electrical meter. Her task is to make her needle follow (or "track") the movements of the other needle which is under automatic control.

where a tracing that had looked like the others now is beginning to increase in amplitude, signifying rising tension in one (and only one) set of muscles: those involved in her complaint (the muscles of the left thigh).

Figure 3.2 is a graphic presentation of the essential facts: when the loud distracting noise was turned on during tracking, tension in the left thigh rose much higher than in the right thigh. Quantitative analysis of simultaneous recordings of tension from other parts of the body (not plotted in the figure) showed that the tension was specific to the left thigh and was not merely increased on the entire left side of the body. The increased tension was specific to the muscle group that had been causing the patient severe discomfort.

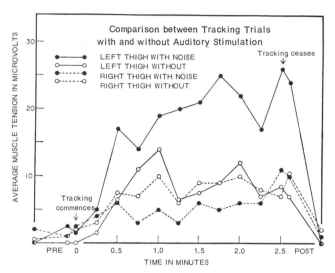

Figure 3.2. *Case 1. Cramping feelings in muscles of left thigh.* Turning on loud noise, while patient is tracking, causes muscle potentials from her left thigh (symptom area) to rise high, far exceeding those for symptom-free right thigh. (Compare two graphs with blackened circles.) When tracking was done under more favorable (distraction-free) conditions, tension in symptom muscle (left thigh) was about the same as tension in the muscles of the right thigh. (Compare two graphs with open circles.) (From Malmo, Activation: A neuropsychological dimension. *Psychological Review*, 1959, *66*, 367–386. Copyright 1959 by the American Psychological Association, and reproduced by permission.)

Case 2.   Painful Tightness on the Right Side of the Neck

This case involves a depressed, unmarried woman of twenty-eight[1] who complained of a painful tightness on the right side of her neck. This symptom had appeared previously, and at the time we made the EMG recordings she had been suffering from this tension for some weeks.

This young woman feared contact with men. This fear may have been caused in part by severe punishment that she received as a child, from her mother who believed that the patient and her brother had been engaging in sex play.

The patient had considered marriage but only under the absurd conditions of agreeing that there would be no sexual intercourse. In fact, she

---

[1] The reader will note that all of the cases described in this chapter are women. This should not be taken to mean that this kind of complaint is more frequent in women than in men. It so happened that at the time these electromyographic recordings were taken the majority of patients in the Institute were women.

stated these conditions to a man who had proposed to her just prior to her coming to our psychiatric Institute.

Considering this fear of contact with men, the results of an unplanned incident during EMG recording are of special interest. The EMG tracings in Figure 3.3 were recorded soon after the patient had finished her tracking test. She was resting quietly while a male research assistant began to remove cloth electrode holders from her arm. In so doing he happened to take her hand in his, whereupon (as Figure 3.3 shows) the EMGs from her right neck muscles suddenly increased in level while, at the same time, the EMGs from the opposite side of her neck showed little or no change. It was established that the rise in right neck muscle tension was not an artifact of head turning or of any other kind of head movement.

Specific   Muscle –Tension   Reaction   in   Symptom   Area

Specific   Muscle –Tension   Reaction   in   Symptom   Area

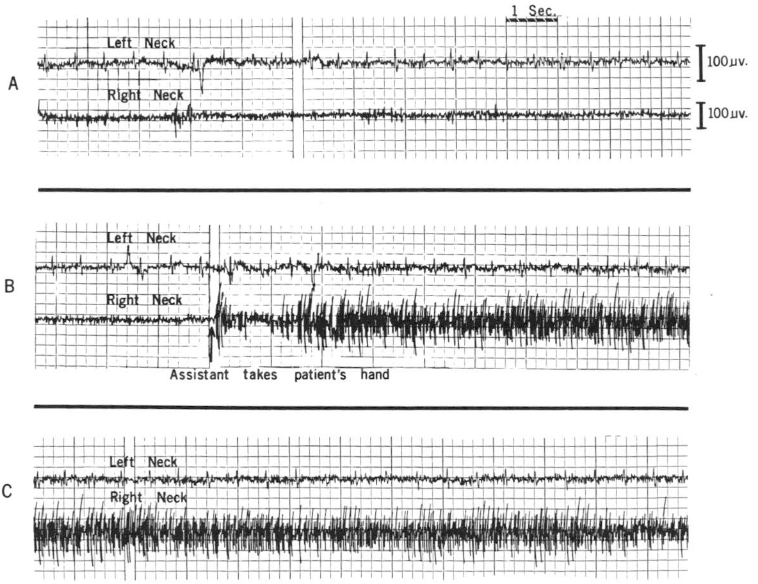

Figure 3.3.   *Case 2. Painful tightness on right side of neck.*   Shy and fearful of men, the patient was evidently embarrassed by the male assistant taking her hand. Note that the muscle-tension reaction to this emotional experience was specific to the muscles involved in her symptom. The EMG reaction was not due to some movement artifact such as head turning. (From unpublished research by R. B. Malmo.)

By taking her hand in his the male assistant evidently embarrassed her by an unintended act of intimacy, at the same time triggering her specific tensional reaction.

EMGs were recorded from this patient while she was being interviewed by her therapist. During the interview, right neck muscle tension rose to more than double left neck tension and to 10–20 times the level of tension in the arm muscles. Again, we observe specific activation of the symptom mechanism, this time in reaction to topics discussed in interview.

This patient also took the tracking test. At the beginning of tracking, right neck tension was much higher than tension recorded from the other muscles. After some minutes of quiet tracking, her neck tension fell gradually. However, like the first patient, she reacted specifically with her symptom-related muscles when the loud distracting sound was turned on. When the noise came on, right neck muscle tension increased markedly, whereas tension in other muscles, including those on the left side of the neck, showed no rise whatever.

At this stage of the case presentations, two points may be made. First, the electromyograms clearly indicated that the source of the patient's discomfort was muscular. This point is proven even more conclusively in some following cases in which rising muscular tension was observed actually to coincide with the patient's complaint of pain during the recording session. Second, there was precise agreement between the specific site of pain and the site from which increased muscular activity was recorded electromyographically. There was thus an objective confirmation of the patient's subjective complaint, which is useful in countering the assertions of unsympathetic relatives and others that "it was all in the patient's mind!"

The reason for individual differences in the specific site of the troublesome muscle group is not very well understood. This is part of a general question that will be discussed in the next chapter.

Here it is relevant to mention some observations from three healthy young men whose EMGs were taken from various muscle groups as they performed in tracking sessions during a 60-hour period of sleep deprivation (Malmo & Surwillo, 1960). Toward the end of this period, for each man there was one muscle group that yielded a decidedly steeper rise during tracking than any other muscle group. Furthermore, the muscle group showing maximal activation differed in each case: one man showed it in the neck, the second in the forehead, and the third in the right biceps muscle.

In short, there were clear individual differences in the site of greatest rise in electromyographic level. This kind of observation is a common one in psychophysiology, following a principle called *physiological response specificity*.

Case 3. "Stiffness" in the Left Side of Neck   This case is an interesting addition to the series because of its complementary relation to the previous one: discomfort from neck muscle tension again, but this time of the left side. Another reason for including this case is that it illustrates the kind of life "stress" that is often associated with the development of chronic anxiety (see previous chapter).

The patient was an attractive twenty-seven-year-old single German girl who for the past two years had been suffering from her tension symptom. She had seen a chiropractor whose treatment had given her only temporary relief. The pain commenced on the left side of her neck, continued down to her left shoulder, and then returned to her head. A headache often developed in this way. The most constant feature of these sensations was "stiffness" in the left side of her neck. This specific symptom was part of a generally overtense attitude which the patient presented.

The patient came to Montreal from Germany five years prior to admission to our psychiatric Institute. She worked first as a hospital attendant and later as a waitress. Being ambitious, she greatly overextended herself by taking a secretarial course in addition to her full-time job as waitress and a part-time evening job as cashier. She was unable to keep up this pace; finding it impossible to concentrate on her work for the course, she finally had to give it up.

She considered herself a failure. For some time she struggled with the conflict between her ambition and her fear of breaking down again. Her long-continued struggle with this conflict, combined with her exhausting work schedule, helped to produce a state of chronic anxiety. Over a period of a year or two, before admission, in addition to the specific tensional symptom, the patient had many of the common symptoms of chronic anxiety, including weight loss, insomnia, and inability to relax.

Electromyographic Investigation   In this case, the specific tensional reaction was activated during the period when she was waiting to have procedures explained to her. For the investigation of her tension symptom we had selected the thermal-pain apparatus, which had been used in our research on anxiety patients (see Chapter II). She was evidently apprehensive about these stimulations, although she was most cooperative. In the pretest period, level of neck muscle tension was clearly higher on the left side (where her symptom was located) than on the right.

Case 4.   Tension in Muscles of the Left Shoulder   When this forty-three-year-old woman was admitted to our psychiatric Institute she was depressed and crying. She complained of pain. She was definite in stating that her left shoulder was the most troublesome tension area. Occasionally there was some discomfort from the right shoulder, but the tensional discomfort was always worse on the left, she said.

The upper electrode of the bipolar pair was placed on the left shoulder at the point where the patient said she felt pain. This seemed to be the focus of pain which radiated downward to the hip region. (The lower electrode was placed nearby.) A bilaterally symmetrical electrode placement was made on the right shoulder.

The technique used with this patient was interview playback. The patient lay in bed listening to the playback of an interview that had been recorded on the previous day. There was one topic in the interview that had made the patient cry. This topic, when played back, again made her cry. It was about the patient's dead sister who had had a difficult life. They had been very close, but at their last meeting, just before her sister died, they had a misunderstanding, which left the patient with a persistent feeling of remorse.

During the playback of this part of the interview, the tension in the left shoulder (which had been at about the same level as tension in the right shoulder) rose to a much higher level. Careful observation of the patient indicated that this tensional rise in the muscles of the left shoulder was not due to bodily movements. Playback is a good arrangement, incidentally, for keeping movements to a minimum because the patient lies quietly in bed listening to the playback, not talking and not moving the hands frequently as in actual interview.

The EMG reaction in this case is especially interesting because the patient stated that tensional discomfort was minimal on the day of the interview playback. In other words, this was "subclinical" activation of the symptom mechanism. That is, the greater proneness of the left shoulder muscles to tension was demonstrated without actually producing the subjective feeling of pain.

We now proceed to two cases where, during interview, tension symptoms were actually elicited, along with corresponding rise in muscle tension seen in the EMG. Tension continued rising during interview (until the patient actually complained of headache).

Strong Activation of Symptom Mechanism during Interview: Continuous Muscle Tension Rise to Level Where Patient Complains of Pain

Case 5. Pain in Back of the Head Mrs. B, a thirty-four-year-old recent widow with anxiety, complained of frequent pain in the back of her head. Her history was one of gross maladjustment extending back to childhood. To all the staff at our psychiatric Institute it was obvious that her hostility was easily aroused. The major event precipitating her breakdown was her husband's fatal accident which occurred soon after she had had a quarrel with him.

EMGs were recorded from Mrs. B while she lay in bed being interviewed by her therapist. Neck electrodes were placed on her symptom area over muscles at the back of her head. There was no pain in that area at the beginning of the interview. For comparison with EMGs from the symptom area, electrodes were also placed on the forehead.

Figure 3.4 shows the course of muscle tension during interview. Dur-

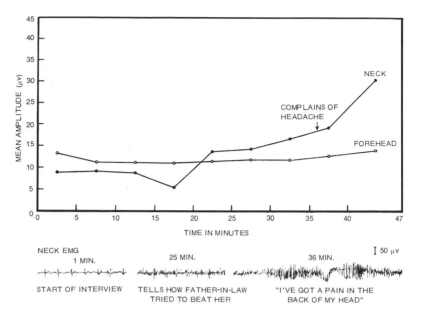

Figure 3.4   *Case 5. Pain in the back of the head.*   The interview begins with relatively indifferent material, and early in the interview neck EMG level is relatively low. As topics in the interview become more emotional in tone, 15–20 minutes after the beginning of the interview, neck tension begins to rise. Failure of curve for forehead tension to rise indicates that in this case it was not all muscles of the head and neck that showed correlation with complaint of headache. Sections of actual neck EMG tracings are shown below the graphs. Mrs. B complains of headache after nearly 20 minutes of steadily rising neck muscle tension (at the 36-minute point in the interview). The topic under discussion prior to Mrs. B's complaint of headache was events leading up to her husband's fatal accident. (After Shagass & Malmo, *Psychodynamic themes and localized muscular tension during psychotherapy. Psychosomatic Medicine*, 1954, *16*, 295–313.)

ing the thirty-sixth minute the patient complained of headache. Her neck EMG for a portion of this minute is reproduced in the figure, along with brief segments of the EMG recording from earlier parts of the interview. The close relation between her subjective complaint of headache, and the objective fact of steadily rising neck muscle tension is clear. The curve for forehead tension, on the other hand, is virtually flat, which is of interest in regard to the next case.

Case 6.   Severe Headaches: Bandlike across the Forehead   Miss A, a forty-five-year-old typist, had strong feelings of inadequacy and insecurity. There was also an undercurrent of hostility, directed mainly toward men. Her therapist found her to be extremely tense and rigid.

Miss A felt so inadequate in trying to talk to another person that conversation was a great strain for her. She was at her most tense when she was trying hard to think of something to say and the words would not come. Associated with these personality weaknesses there were a number of bodily complaints, the most troublesome one being severe headaches, bandlike across the forehead. Miss A reported that these headaches seemed to wax and wane according to the intensity of stresses that she encountered.

EMG Recording during Interview   EMGs from Miss A's forehead and right forearm were recorded in twelve interviews conducted while the patient lay on a bed in the experimental room. The tape recording of interview content was synchronized with the EMG tracings (see Davis & Malmo, 1951).

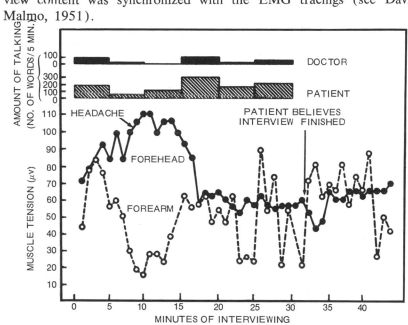

Figure 3.5   *Case 6. Bandlike headaches across forehead.*   Miss A complains of headache during the interview at the point shown in graph. Miss A is under stress at this point because her therapist is forcing her to take the initiative; he is trying unsuccessfully to get her to produce meaningful topics for discussion. During the first five minutes, her doctor explained how he wanted the interview to be conducted, and Miss A asked him questions about the procedure. In the second five minutes, the doctor says as little as he can (notice drop in his amount of talking shown in bar graph); but Miss A is still unproductive. She talks less and less, and what she does say is superficial and repetitious. Forehead muscle EMG *rises*. *Forearm* muscle EMG *falls* during this period probably because with less and less talking Miss A's habitual use of hands during talking is reduced more and more. When the doctor resumes his supportive role, forehead muscle EMG falls and forearm muscle EMG rises. Later in the interview when the patient believes the interview is finished, her forehead muscle EMG drops and then rises again when she realizes the interview will continue. (From Davis & Malmo, *American Journal of Psychiatry*, 1951, *107*, 908–916. Copyright 1951, the American Psychiatric Association.)

The seventh interview was conducted in a special way. Soon after the beginning of the interview, the therapist put the patient much more on her own than hitherto. Because of Miss A's difficulty in communicating, he realized that forcing her to take initiative for the material to be discussed would be tension-producing. But he hoped that this experience might help the patient to work better in psychotherapy.

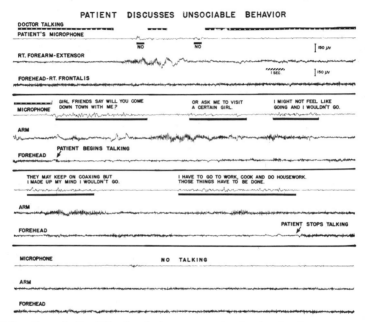

Figure 3.6.   *Case 6. Bandlike headaches across forehead.*   EMGs recorded from Miss A during interview show: Talking, which relieves emotional strain, reduces forehead muscle tension. Output from the patient's microphone also is recorded on paper. When the patient talks, pickup from the microphone causes deflections to appear on the record. These deflections have been underlined on the record, and what Miss A said each time has been printed in above. Find the beginning of the tracing labeled "forehead-rt. frontalis." This is the EMG for the forehead muscle. (*Frontalis* is the technical term and "rt." refers to the fact that the electrodes were placed to right of center.) After this, the continuations of the EMG recordings from the forehead are labeled simply "forehead." The continuous EMG recording has been cut into four strips. In the part of the interview corresponding to the first strip, Miss A spoke only two words, and evidently this was insufficient to reduce forehead muscle tension. Near the beginning of the second strip of forehead EMG, arrow marks point where the patient begins talking. The EMG tracing immediately becomes thinner, indicating decrease in forehead muscle tension. Now drop down to the third strip where near the end, arrow marks point where the patient stops talking. The immediate thickening of the tracing (that is, higher EMG level) at this point is obvious. EMG showed that forehead muscle tension remained at this higher level throughout the fourth strip at the bottom of the figure. During this entire period of higher forehead muscle tension Miss A was silent. EMGs from right forearm indicated that Miss A used her right hand while talking. (From Davis & Malmo, *American Journal of Psychiatry,* 1951, *107,* 908–916. Copyright 1951, the American Psychiatric Association.)

Figure 3.5 shows the effects of this procedure on the EMGs. Forehead muscle tension climbed high, and as it was reaching a peak (after about 8½ minutes of this special session), Miss A spontaneously complained of headache.

When the doctor resumed his usual supportive role, Miss A's forehead tension dropped, despite the fact that she was talking more.

Like Mrs. B, Miss A's EMGs furnished clear objective evidence that strong activation of a specific muscle group was associated with her headaches. Different emotions were associated with the headaches in the two cases (and of course different muscle groups as well).

As previously explained, Miss A was under great strain when she could think of nothing worthwhile to say; and when at last she found something to say, the strain was relieved temporarily. These rises and falls in emotional strain were reflected in her forehead EMGs recorded during interview. During silent periods her forehead muscle tension rose; when she began talking, it fell (see Figure 3.6). There was a remarkable consistency in this. Only seven times in 465 measurements were there *increases* of forehead tension with talking! This is all the more remarkable because in normal persons the very activity of talking causes forehead muscle tension to *increase*. The keys to understanding these remarkable findings are (a) the specific reaction of Miss A's forehead muscle tension to the emotion-producing situation, and (b) the extraordinarily high background level of forehead muscle tension, which being so high, could readily come down when anything happened to reduce emotional strain.

Miss A's forehead muscle tension in her early interviews rose to

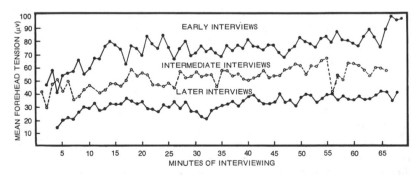

Figure 3.7. *Case 6. Bandlike headaches across forehead.* Forehead muscle EMGs show reduction in tension over a series of interviews. Each graph shows minute-by-minute forehead muscle tension plotted from averages of three interviews: (a) early, (b) in the middle of the series, and (c) later. Miss A reported headaches toward the end of the early interviews when forehead muscle tension had risen to high levels. (From Davis & Malmo, *American Journal of Psychiatry*, 1951, *107*, 908–916. Copyright 1951, the American Psychiatric Association.)

nearly 100 microvolts (see Figure 3.7), high enough to give her headaches (which she reported). In later interviews, average tension level had dropped to about half the initial level, and headaches were not reported.

On the Treatment of Severe Chronic Tension Headaches

According to neurologist J. Edmeads the so-called muscle relaxant drugs when taken by mouth "have very little muscle relaxant action, and it is only when they are given intravenously in large doses that they have demonstrable effect in reducing the . . . E.M.G. potentials of muscles in spasm (Edmeads, 1971, p. 38)." However, as Edmeads explains, in many patients these drugs when taken orally do relieve headaches, but in indirect ways which are not well understood.

On the basis of his experience as a practicing neurologist, Edmeads (1971) believes that this kind of headache is generally closely associated with what he refers to as "emotional tension." Edmeads discusses various kinds of headaches. In this chapter we have seen examples of how certain "emotionally toned" situations were indeed associated with rising muscle tension, which was specifically localized in the symptom area. A recent development, that of feedback treatment of tension headaches, will be described in Chapter IV.

PERVASIVENESS OF MUSCLE TENSION RISES IN A WIDE VARIETY OF PSYCHOLOGICAL FUNCTIONS: MUSCLE TENSION GRADIENTS

The rising EMG curve from the first (stressful) part of Miss A's interview (see Figure 3.5) represents a special instance of an extremely pervasive phenomenon: the electromyographic (EMG) gradient.

The term *EMG gradients* applies to a progressively rising level of voltage, which reflects gradually rising tension in the specific muscle group on which the electrodes are placed (refer back to Chapter I). The lower part of Figure 3.4 presents three strips of "raw" EMG tracings, illustrating the incremental change in neck EMG amplitude during an interview. The curve for neck muscle EMG in the upper part of Figure 3.4 is plotted from successive measurements of EMG level. This represents the basic method used in plotting EMG gradients. Before proceeding to further examples of these EMG gradients, it will be helpful to make a few general statements about them. They appear only in certain muscles. We have previously noted individual differences in this respect. There are also situational differences. For example, during tracking with the right arm, EMG gradients are prominent in recordings from the nontracking left forearm muscles, whereas, as we shall see presently, listening attentively to a story usually results in EMG gradients being recorded from the muscles of the forehead. Steepness of the gradient is a significant feature. Generally speaking, the stronger the person's involvement in what he or she is doing, the steeper the gradient. Various examples of this will be given later in this chapter. The correct way to view the gradient is to regard the *steepness* of rise throughout the entire course of the sequence (for example, story listened to, tracking trial, interview) as an index of involvement in the whole sequence from beginning to end. From our observations (to be discussed later) we know that it is wrong to interpret the rising tension simply as the person's involvement increasing more and more *during* the sequence. This statement may seem puzzling. However, if the reader will accept this statement on faith now, it will be useful in the following discussion. Later in this chapter (and again in Chapter V), the reasons for this statement will be discussed in detail.

As the reader has gathered from these general remarks, EMG gradients appear in situations where persons are not required to move any muscles; and similar gradients also appear in situations that do require some coordinated muscular effort, like rotating a knob in a tracking skill. In the psychological sense, both kinds of activity require *effort* and, as previously suggested, EMG gradients reflect degree of effort (or of *involvement*). This observation is useful in exposing the artificiality of hard and fast distinctions between "mental activity" and "motor acts."

In addition to their indicating degree of psychological involvement (or effort), EMG gradients appear to be related to another equally important neuropsychological function. This is the brain mechanism that keeps a behavior sequence going from beginning to end. In telling a story, for instance, one is not merely led along sentence by sentence, as one would have to be in finding the way along a chain link by link in the dark. Instead, the whole story, consisting of main points leading up to the climax or punch line, is kept in mind throughout. There must be a fairly high-level mechanism in the brain that provides for overall continuity—an organizing function that is distinct from the more mechanical ones. An analogy in music would be the composer's overall conception of a new symphony on the one hand, and his setting down the notes for the instruments in the orchestra on the other. The fact that EMG gradients usually fail to appear with psychologically low-level repetitive types of activity (for example, simple tapping on a telegraph key) suggests that when EMG gradients do occur they are related to some brain mechanism responsible for high-level sequential organization.

Examples of EMG Gradients

EMG Gradients during Listening to Recorded Stories   Figure 3.8 presents the main results of an experiment by Wallerstein (1954) in our laboratory. His subjects were men who lay comfortably on a bed, listening to a good

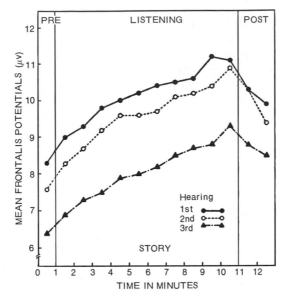

Figure 3.8 *Effect of listening to a detective story on forehead muscle tension.* The person reclines comfortably, enjoying a detective story played to him on a tape recorder. Muscle potentials are recorded from the forehead. During listening muscle tension climbs steadily, and at the end tension falls. Graphs are based on averages from nineteen men, who listened to the same story three times. Forehead tension rose every time, but level of tension dropped each time the story was repeated. (From Wallerstein, An electromyographic study of attentive listening. *Canadian Journal of Psychology*, 1954, *8*, 228–238.)

detective story played on a tape recorder. The figure shows the EMG gradients associated with listening to the story. It is of interest to note that the highest average level of muscle tension reached was only about one-tenth that of Miss A's in the stressful interview (Figure 3.5). It is important always to distinguish between the *absolute EMG level* reached and the *steepness of the gradient*. The extremely high level of the former in Miss A's case is significant in relation to her complaint of headache.

Again in our laboratory, Bartoshuk (1956) repeated this experiment, using the same story, and once more observed EMG gradients. He also obtained some data bearing directly on the relation between gradient steepness and involvement in listening. He found that the EMG gradients of listeners who rated their stories high in interest value were generally steeper than gradients of listeners who gave lower ratings to the story.

In addition, Bartoshuk recorded from the brain, using an electroencephalograph (EEG). A brief explanation of certain EEG phenomena will assist the reader in understanding the relations between EEG and EMG that Bartoshuk found.

Look at the bottom four tracings (E–H) in Figure 3.9; and compare

BILATERAL PARIETAL EEG

SUBJECTS WITH POSITIVE FRONTALIS EMG GRADIENTS

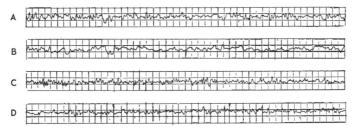

SUBJECTS WITH NEGATIVE FRONTALIS EMG GRADIENTS

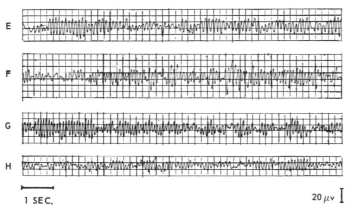

1 SEC.   20 μν

Figure 3.9 *Samples of electroencephalograms (EEGs) from eight different persons who later listened to a 10-minute detective story.* Top four ("beta") EEG tracings (A–D) are typical of persons who are either involved or preparing to be engaged in tasks requiring sustained attention. During listening, forehead EMGs of these persons showed gradients. Bottom four EEG tracings (E–H) are typical of very relaxed, relatively uninvolved state (lower frequency, higher amplitude of waves). In these persons, rising EMG gradients failed to appear during playing of record.

EEG electrodes were in the parietal region, being placed about two-thirds of the distance from the bridge of the nose to the bony prominence (*inion*) at the back of head. (From Bartoshuk, EMG gradients and EEG amplitude during motivated listening. *Canadian Journal of Psychology*, 1956, *10*, 156–164.)

them with the top four tracings (A–D). Note in the bottom tracings that there are about 8–12 waves per second. These frequencies, which are in the *alpha* range, are generally recorded from persons who are relaxed and relatively uninvolved in anything requiring sustained attention. On the other hand, the four top tracings (A–D) are typical of EEG recordings from persons who are either involved or preparing to be engaged in some task requiring sustained attention. These *beta* waves are of lower amplitude and there are more of them per second than in the case of the alpha waves. Change from alpha to beta EEG usually signifies a change from relaxed wakefulness to a state of attentive involvement in some activity, or preparation to engage in some activity. It is interesting, therefore, that Bartoshuk recorded good EMG gradients from persons who had the beta EEG pattern prior to listening to the story, and that he failed to obtain EMG gradients from persons who had the alpha EEG pattern beforehand.[2]

It is also important (though not surprising) to note that there were no EEG gradients going along with the EMG gradients. The same conclusion (that is, no EEG gradients accompanying EMG gradients) was drawn from some experiments with tracking to which we now turn.

EMG Gradients during Tracking   Figure 3.10 presents averaged EMG gradients recorded from the muscles of the left forearms of men using their right hands in tracking. We obtained the data shown in the figure by using a tracking apparatus. The tracking task was similar to the one previously described: the person rotated a knob slowly back and forth with his right hand. However, instead of being guided by a moving meter needle as before, the person was guided by tones heard in earphones. When he turned the knob at precisely the correct velocity, the person heard no tone in his earphones. When the velocity of rotation exceeded

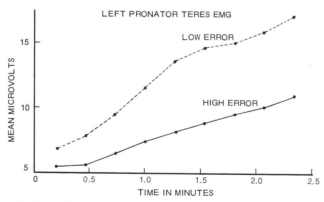

Figure 3.10   *EMG gradients from muscles of the left forearm during tracking with right hand.*   The steeper gradient was obtained from averaged EMGs recorded during the best trial (that is, the one with the lowest error score) in each case. The less steep gradient was obtained from trial with highest error score (poorest performance). (From Malmo, Physiological gradients and behavior. *Psychological Bulletin*, 1965, *64*, 225–234. Copyright 1965 by the American Psychological Association, and reproduced by permission.)

[2] Because of its regular sine-wave appearance, alpha EEG is sometimes referred to as *synchronized*, in contrast with beta, which is referred to as *desynchronized*. The latter is also referred to as *low voltage, fast frequency waves*.

this value, he heard a tone in one of the earphones (in the right earphone during clockwise rotation and in the left earphone during counterclockwise rotation). Conversely, when the velocity of rotation lagged behind the correct value, he heard a tone in the opposite earphone (in the left earphone during clockwise rotation and in the right earphone during counterclockwise rotation). The loudness of the tone informed the person about the magnitude of his error from moment to moment.

Figure 3.10 shows that superior (and presumably more highly motivated) tracking and steeper EMG gradients go together. This is further evidence that rising muscle tension in a goal-directed activity has motivational significance.

Figure 3.11 presents data for heart rate and respiration. There is an obvious similarity between the gradients for these autonomic functions and the gradients for muscle tension. It seems reasonable to consider that

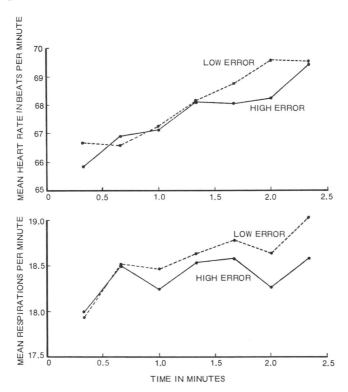

Figure 3.11 *Gradient curves for heart rate and breathing rate.*   Note that, as in the case of muscle potentials, gradients were steeper for better tracking performance. (From Malmo, Physiological gradients and behavior. *Psychological Bulletin*, 1965, *64*, 225–234. Copyright 1965 by the American Psychological Association, and reproduced by permission.)

gradients in heart rate and respiration reflect the usual energizing support of skeletal muscle activity by autonomic nervous system mechanisms, which provide more blood for the muscles and in general provide favorable conditions (such as increased oxygen supply) for facilitating muscular contractions.

Figure 3.12 presents EEG data which, as in the case of Bartoshuk's experiment, show absence of gradients in EEG during periods when EMGs were showing gradients. The data presented are from the beta EEG band. Analysis of alpha EEG for the same periods also failed to show gradients, or any other progressive change.

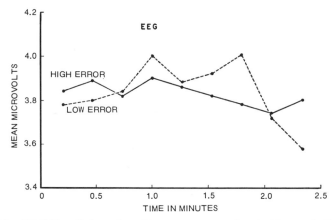

Figure 3.12 *EEG "beta" data plotted in same way as data in Figures 3.10 and 3.11.* Comparisons show that EEG graphs are different: No gradients appear. See text for further details concerning analysis of EEG data. (From Malmo, Physiological gradients and behavior. *Psychological Bulletin*, 1965, *64*, 225–234. Copyright 1965 by the American Psychological Association, and reproduced by permission.)

Figure 3.13 shows performance scores plotted in such a way that comparisons may be made with the curves for EMG, heart rate, respiration, and EEG. Note that in common with the EEG curves in the preceding figure, these curves for performance show no regularly rising gradients.

Observe, for example, the contrast between the regularly rising EMG gradients in Figure 3.10 and the graphs in Figures 3.12 and 3.13, which show no gradients. The sudden rises in error appearing in the graphs for performance in Figure 3.13 can be accounted for by reference to the physical conditions of the task. These were the places in the tracking where the person was required to reverse direction in rotating the tracking knob (from counterclockwise to clockwise). It is clear from these data that the EMG gradients represent rising muscle tension accompanying relatively constant performance.

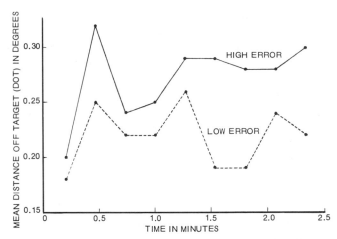

Figure 3.13   *Performance data from tracking task plotted so that they may be compared with EMG gradients in Figure 3.10.*   Graphs reflect relatively even performance throughout tracking trial, with periodic rises in error score due to the person's having to reverse direction of tracking knob at these particular times. Contrast these graphs with the evenly progressive curves for muscle tension (that is, EMG gradients) in Figure 3.10. (From Malmo, Physiological gradients and behavior. *Psychological Bulletin*, 1965, *64*, 225–234. Copyright 1965 by the American Psychological Association, and reproduced by permission.)

On the Interpretation of EMG Gradients

At this point in the review of the empirical findings, it should be useful to discuss some general points concerning the interpretation of EMG gradients. The EMG gradient appears to be reflecting the operation of some complex central mechanism, which plays a role in sustaining a behavior sequence (such as performing a task or attending to a story). According to the evidence from the EMG gradients, one likely feature of this central mechanism seems to be a positively accelerating output to certain muscles, which is observed under conditions of fairly regular, even performance throughout a continuous behavioral sequence. The evidence from the experiments suggests a hypothetical *central* mechanism going faster and faster throughout the behavior sequence and, we think, having something to do with producing continuous unflagging performance. In relating the hypothetical "gradient mechanism" to performance level, an image that comes to mind is Alice and the Red Queen of Looking-Glass Land, having to run faster and faster in order to stay in the same place.

However, as should be clear by now, the claim is *not* made that rising muscle tension per se does anything, necessarily. Our evidence for the hypothetical central mechanism is admittedly indirect. We stress the point that we are talking about co-occurring events. However, the correlations are strengthened by the relatively large number of observations revealing EMG gradients present in a wide variety of situations.[3]

To repeat, the hypothesis is that gradients reflect central mechanisms mediating various kinds of purposive, goal-directed behavioral sequences, demarcating beginning and end of each sequence. The pervasiveness of EMG gradients over a wide range of behavioral sequences makes this an attractive hypothesis. In other words, according to the hypothesis, the appearance of a gradient indicates the occurrence of an organized behavior sequence. This is the first point. The second point is that the *rate* of muscle-tension increase (that is, steepness of the gradient) reflects what we may call (in general terms) degree of involvement.[4]

Decision Making and EMG Gradients   With these working hypotheses in mind, let us review the results of some more experiments. In a study by Bélanger (1957), two tasks were precisely matched for muscular exertion, yet one task produced EMG gradients while the other failed to do so.

Bélanger's subjects, in a task requiring a series of rapid decisions concerning which of six circles projected on a screen was the largest, were required to press a button with their index fingers each time a decision was made. (Each set of circles was projected for only a few seconds.) Bélanger observed EMG gradients within a series of decisions. When the person merely had to press the button at the same intervals *without* being required to make any decisions, no EMG gradients appeared.

Interest Value of Material and EMG Gradients   Wallerstein (1954), it will be recalled, found steep gradients in forehead muscles of subjects listening to a detective story. Also, he observed that persons listening to a less immediately absorbing piece (an excerpt from a philosophical essay) did not show such steep gradients at first, but as they became more interested on repeated presentations, the gradients became steeper.

In other experiments from our laboratory, we observed that when persons were "turned off" during listening to a poor recording of a boring article, their EMGs stopped climbing and began to fall.

Perhaps some time in the future, some lazy dramatic critic may wish to dispense with writing reviews, and to substitute ratings based on his EMG gradients fed into a computer for analysis and printout! (Objections could certainly be anticipated!) Facetiousness aside, the technique does indeed seem promising for the objective monitoring of duration and intensity of sequential covert silent activity (such as thought).

---

[3] The reader who is interested in this literature may consult Malmo (1965) for a summary and for references to the original articles.

[4] Some psychologists (followers of C. L. Hull) might be inclined to view *steepness* of EMG gradients as reflecting relative strength of anticipatory goal responses.

Hallucinations and EMG Gradients   There are other forms of covert silent activity (rather mysterious ones) that EMG recordings might help to elucidate: for instance, *hallucinations* (to use the conventional clinical term for "hearing imaginary voices"). We were fortunate to find a cooperative patient who was willing to work with us in our efforts to determine whether EMG gradients might accompany hallucinatory sequences.

Our patient was a twenty-seven-year-old man. One month prior to our EMG recording, he had been acutely confused, with complaints of insomnia and aching pains over his body. He said that he heard voices. This patient appeared especially well suited for our experiment because of his cooperativeness, and also because of his own observations concerning his hallucinations.

He described the "voices" as coming on after his own tongue and lips had moved; and interestingly, he stated the voices would cease if someone talked to him. Accordingly, we arranged with the patient's doctor to have chin EMGs recorded in a situation conducive to hallucinations (that is, in a quiet room with the doctor present but not speaking), and after a period of hallucinating to have his doctor commence talking to the patient in order to make the hallucination cease.

The patient indicated by button pressures when the hallucinatory sequences began and when they ceased. In addition to EMG recording from his chin, EMGs were also recorded from his left forearm extensor muscles. We had earlier determined in a number of other experiments that EMG recordings from the chin mainly reflected activity of the speech muscles.

The results of this experiment are shown in Figure 3.14. The figure shows the integrated EMGs that were recorded continuously throughout two hallucinatory periods. Each spike-shaped deflection in the record represents the average muscle tension for a 4-second period. Look first at the left end of the top line labeled "chin." Note that the tops of the first deflections barely reach, or do not quite reach, the nearest grid line. Now moving from left to right, note that the deflections rise above this line, and toward the end of the tracing nearly reach the next grid line above. This is typical of an EMG gradient, as is the drop in EMG level when the gradient is completed. In this case, the drop in tension was preceded by a burst of EMG activity, which occurred following the doctor's interruption.

Now look at the line marked "left forearm extensor" in the top tracing and note that the deflections do not change during the hallucination. Now examine the lower part of the figure, which shows the EMG integrator tracings from the second hallucinatory period. Look first at the tracing for the chin muscle. Note that the deflections at the end of the hallucinatory period are three to four times higher than those at the

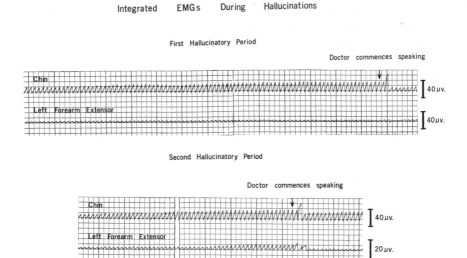

Figure 3.14. *EMG gradients in integrated recordings from speech muscles (chin electrodes) during two hallucinatory periods.* Muscle potentials from forearm also show EMG gradient in the second period. Each integration period was four seconds: First hallucinatory period was about six minutes; second period was about 3½ minutes. (See text for explanation.) (From unpublished research by R. B. Malmo.)

beginning. This degree of increment in muscle tension is somewhat greater than it was for the first hallucinatory period (that is, the steepness of the EMG gradient was greater). Note further that for the second hallucinatory period the integrator tracing for the left forearm extensor also shows a gradient, although the level of muscle tension is only about one-fourth that of the chin muscle tension. The fact that the chin EMG showed a gradient both times and that the forearm EMG showed a gradient only once is of interest. Our sample is too small to justify much comment. However, we would expect EMG gradients to appear more consistently in recordings from the speech muscles because of their presumed primary relation to hallucinations; and occasional gradients from additional muscles is a common finding (see Malmo, 1965, for further details). The pattern of tensional changes in the chin muscles corresponded well with the patient's own description of the pattern of hallucinatory activity characteristic for him, and with the patient's statements to the doctor after the recording session in our laboratory. The patient stated that he gradually became aware of "voices" soon after the room was quiet, and ceased hearing the voices during the time the doctor was talking to him. Then, after her talking ceased, he gradually became aware of "the voices" again.

The EMG gradients and the patient's preoccupied behavior during hallucinatory periods suggested that the patient was engaged in organized and absorbing mental activity. The EMG gradients contributed valuable information because, as expected, the patient either could not recall or chose not to report the content of his hallucinations. During the session, when she interrupted the patient's hallucinations, the doctor chose geographical (nonemotional) topics to talk about. The patient's recall of what the doctor had said was good, but he insisted that he had "forgotten what the voices said." It has been found that many "hallucinators" are reluctant to discuss their imaginings (Weiner, 1967).

Jonathan Lang, one of the few schizophrenics ever to write lucidly about his psychosis, said that sometimes his hallucinations took the form of short playlets (Lang, 1939). Further study of hallucinations, using the EMG technique, appears promising for enriching knowledge about this fascinating and mysterious form of silent covert activity.

Dreams and EMG Gradients   While few of us have ever experienced hallucinations (for example, "heard voices" when no one was speaking), all of us have had dreams. The possibility of EMG gradients being associated with dream sequences in sleep was suggested to me by D. O. Hebb (1967, p. 315).

Most sleep researchers have employed EMGs sparingly, if at all. Some have used only one channel of EMG recording (for example, from neck muscles), and have relatively neglected the other possible contributions of electromyography. However, McGuigan and Tanner (1971) have demonstrated the usefulness of lip and chin EMGs in the study of dreaming.

In our laboratory, in the few EMGs that we have recorded during sleep, we have actually seen EMG gradients; so we know they can occur despite the obvious fact that muscle activity is very low during sleep. From the appearance of the records, these gradients seemed to occur in the absence of gross bodily movent. Furthermore, as previously explained, other physiological functions show gradients, and they may yield useful additional information in sleep research.

Dream Recall   Now a brief digression is in order to call attention to an important phenomenon of dream recall that seems to have escaped the attention of dream researchers. Apparently, it is a fairly common experience that a dream from the previous night is suddenly recalled, usually in the morning within an hour or so after waking, if the person happens to have a perception (or thought) related to the dream. For example, dreams of smoking occur in many persons who have given it up. Recall of a dream about smoking may occur as the person sees a cigarette advertisement on a billboard as he is driving to work. Such recall is of interest because it suggests a kind of bridge between sleeping and waking life. This kind of dream recall, triggered by a stimulus encountered in waking life, although apparently fairly common, is rarely referred to by those investigating dreaming. Some persons, incidentally, who were unaware of having had this experience, when I first asked them about it, later reported dream recall on the basis of such cues.

This kind of dream recall seems to have potential methodological usefulness, as well as being important for theories concerned with dreaming. Many of our dreams are probably forgotten simply because of dissociations between sleeping and waking life, rather than being due entirely (or even mainly) to repressive forces actively blocking the recall of "painful" thoughts (which, as psychoanalytic theory suggests, undoubtedly accounts for *some* forgetting of dreams). Could it not be that during free associations on the analyst's couch, the person might be more likely to turn up an image or a thought that had some connection with a dream the night before than if he had not engaged in the free association procedure? Try recalling dreams on the way to work, and if you find that your dream recall is assisted by things you see, or do, or think about, consider that these perceptions may be regarded as "bridges" across to fragments of your dream life.

Goal Directed Behavior, Involvement, and EMG Gradients   Present-day behavior theorists all seem agreed that stimuli and responses should be seen as inextricably tied together: two continuously interacting factors in a continuous process. The person performing a tracking task, for example, turns the knob while listening to the tones that inform him moment-to-moment how to proceed.

The tracker has an expectation of about how long he must work at the task before a rest period (that is, how long the tracking trial will be). This sets a goal, and the tracking trial may be regarded as a continuous progression toward this goal. This kind of continuous sequence is a universal characteristic of all animal behavior.

Basically, the same kind of progression is characteristic also of thinking and other muted or silent activities. As we have observed previously, (a) the presence of gradients generally signifies the presence of a goal-directed behavior sequence, and (b) gradient steepness is correlated with degree of involvement.

THE MOTOR SYSTEM

Two Kinds of Muscle Fiber

When we attach EMG electrodes to muscles, we are tapping in on the motor system. It would be impossible to overstate the complexity of this system. (As we shall see in a moment, it probably involves the entire brain.) But it should be worthwhile for us to try to understand in very general terms how EMG gradients may be generated, and what significance they may have for the brain and behavior.

As explained in Chapter I, the physical source of muscle potentials is well understood. It is the self-propagating electrical impulse, sweeping over the entire muscle fiber, which causes electrical activity to spread from muscle to skin, where the EMG electrodes pick up the signals that are amplified and recorded as EMGs. The gradual, even rise of muscle potentials (that is, the EMG gradient) is produced by the progressive recruitment of more and more depolarized muscle fibers, causing more and more electrical activity to spread from the muscles to the skin.

Electrical activity is recorded from two kinds of muscle fibers. Look first at Figure 3.15A, which is a diagram illustrating the contraction (shortening) of a muscle fiber and the consequent movement of the bones (assuming that a sufficient number of muscle fibers have contracted). A real muscle fiber is only about one-tenth of a millimeter in diameter, but is often several centimeters long. A muscle may contain tens of thousands of muscle fibers.

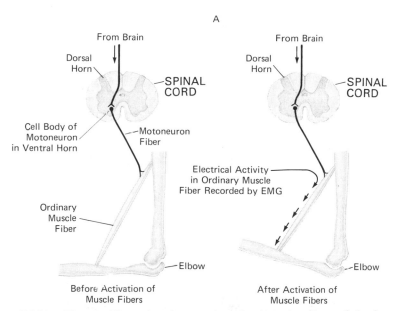

A

Figure 3.15A *Diagram illustrating the neural mechanism of ordinary skeletal muscle contraction.* Motoneuron in spinal cord is fired by nerve endings from cells originating in the brain. Motoneuron in turn stimulates muscle fiber causing it to contract (shorten). Electrical activity that sweeps down muscle fibers during contraction is the source of EMG voltage. Muscle fiber illustrated in this figure is the *ordinary* kind, which in concert with many other fibers of *skeletal* muscle serves to move bony levers. (Adapted from "How we control the contraction of our muscles" by P. A. Merton. Copyright © 1972 by Scientific American, Inc. All rights reserved.)

Next look at Figure 3.15B, which illustrates a second kind of muscle fiber (sometimes referred to as a *modified* muscle fiber). The capsule in the center of this fiber is called the *equatorial capsule* and it contains sensory endings that are wrapped around the muscle fibers. This muscle fiber also contracts (shortens) except for the central part (capsule) containing the sensory endings. The modified muscle fiber receives its own nerve fibers (sometimes called "gamma") and when stimulated by its nerve fibers the modified muscle fiber contracts at both ends (but not in the middle). Since the central capsule does *not* contract, it is pulled (stretched) by the contraction of the fiber on both sides of it. This stretching has the effect of stimulating the sensory fibers (called *stretch receptors*), which in turn causes neural impulses to be carried via the sensory nerve into the spinal cord. While this sensory input plays an important role in spinal reflexes, it is known that neural impulses initiated by these stretch

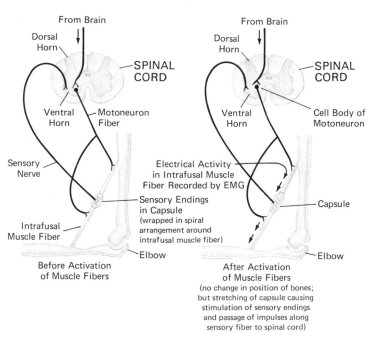

Figure 3.15B *Diagram illustrating the neural mechanism associated with the contraction of modified (intrafusal) muscle fiber, which contracts but does not exert any force on bones.* Instead, the contraction at both ends of the fiber serves to stretch the encapsulated noncontractile middle section, which contains sensory endings. As in the case of the ordinary muscle fibers, their contraction provides a source of voltage that is recorded in the EMG. But the increase in EMG level from this source is independent of skeletal movement (that is, movement of the bones at their joints). (Adapted from "How we control the contraction of our muscles" by P. A. Merton. Copyright © 1972 by Scientific American, Inc. All rights reserved.)

receptors may reach the cerebral cortex. These modified muscle fibers with the sensory endings wrapped around their middle parts (in the capsules) are themselves encased in a sheath or "bag," which is shaped like a spindle (being long and thin and having pointed ends). In fact these "bags" are called *muscle spindles*. Each muscle spindle contains a bundle of the modified muscle fibers, which are called *intrafusal muscle fibers* (from the Latin *fusus*, meaning spindle: *intrafusal* literally means "inside a spindle"). A muscle contains hundreds of spindles which lie among the ordinary muscle fibers (the much longer red stringy structures that actually do the work), and the muscle spindles share with the ordinary muscle fibers the attachments to bone or tendon. However, having their own motor nerve fibers, the intrafusal fibers can be activated while the ordinary muscle fibers remain inactive (and vice versa). We have some evidence from our laboratory that EMG gradients may sometimes, at least, be largely a function of activated *intrafusal* muscle fibers. In tracking, the actual force applied to the knob (as recorded by means of a strain gauge) failed to show a gradient despite the fact that good gradients appeared in the EMGs from the arm muscles. Since the *ordinary* muscle fibers do the actual work (that is, produce the force that is picked up by a strain gauge), the rising gradients could not be attributed to ordinary muscle fibers. Therefore, it seems likely that in this instance, at least, the rising muscle potentials were produced by rising electrical activity that was generated by recruitment of more and more depolarized *intrafusal* fibers.

The sensory fibers going from the sensory endings in the capsule along the sensory nerve fiber to the spinal cord (with connections also to higher brain centers) serve in feedback loops for purposes of motor coordination. They do not enable us to feel the tension in our muscles. There are receptors in the tendons (attachments between muscle and bone) that signal to the nervous system the tension in the part of the muscle in which they lie. Their sensory fibers enter the *dorsal* horn of the spinal cord (see Figure 3.15B). These sense organs (through their functioning to alter action patterns of neurons in the brain) are involved in the discomforts complained of by people with tension symptoms. Sensation at extreme intensity can be uncomfortable even though the person may say that the sensation "isn't exactly one of pain." However, as the intensity increases more and more, a point is reached when most persons will say they "feel pain." From this statement it should not be inferred that pain is merely due to excessive stimulation of any sense organ. Pain is exceedingly complex and a general discussion of the subject is beyond the scope of this book. We shall confine our attention to pains associated with electromyographically recorded high-level muscle tension. Drawing on other recent developments in pain research (Melzack, 1973), two points may be made. First, it should be borne in mind that we are never aware of receptor activity as such. Sensation depends on *patterns* in the brain (which *involve* inputs from receptors). Second, excessive muscle tension is noxious (in at least some instances) because it is injurious to tissue. Under these conditions there is an increase in the activation of *slow conducting sensory fibers* (C fibers) so that the ratio of slow conducting to fast conducting (A) fibers entering the spinal cord is increased. According to the "gate-control" theory, this shift in the C/A ratio opens a "gating" mechanism in the spinal cord, which in turn increases the firing level of certain cells in the dorsal horn of the spinal cord. When their integrated firing level reaches a critical point, these cells (called *T-cells* for "transmission") trigger the brain action system that is responsible for pain experience and response (Melzack, 1973, p. 162).

As Melzack explains, the action system responsible for pain experience and response involves the whole brain, and the key role of the motor system is stressed particularly.

The Motor System: Convergence of Pathways on the Motoneuron in the Spinal Cord

The starting point for this brief description of the motor system is the cell body of the motoneuron lying in the ventral horn of the spinal cord (see Figure 3.15B). We have noted what happens when this cell body is fired on from above. Now we will consider the sources of this supra-spinal stimulation of the motoneuron.

First of all, the single input from the brain shown in Figure 3.15 is a gross oversimplification. Actually there is a convergence on the moto-neuron from some seven or more different brain areas. The reader must bear in mind that when we speak of the *motor system* we are referring to a highly complex system involving many brain areas. However, it is a relatively well-defined system in the sense that it is comprised of brain structures that project *directly* to the motoneurons in the ventral horns of the spinal cord (and to the motor nuclei of the cranial nerves). In addition to being influenced in its firing pattern by this convergence of pathways from the brain, the motoneuron for an ordinary muscle fiber may be fired at the spinal level by sensory fibers from the sensory endings in the capsule of an intrafusal muscle fiber. In Figure 3.15B the motoneuron cell body, its axon, and the ordinary muscle fiber were omitted for sake of simplicity. But the reader may sketch them in by placing the symbol for a cell body (•) inside the V-shaped symbol for the axon terminal left open in Figure 3.15B. When these structures are diagrammed in, the feedback loop of the stretch reflex is completed. Firing the motoneuron for the ordinary muscle fiber can then occur either when the muscle is stretched mechanically or when the motoneuron for the intrafusal muscle fiber is stimulated through one or more of the pathways descending from the brain. The latter sequence possibly provides a feedforward mechanism, like power steering in an automobile (Merton, 1972). Contraction of the intrafusal muscle fibers could in effect drive the ordinary muscle fibers by means of the stretch reflex, bringing more of them into contraction at the proper time to ensure good muscular coordination and, vice versa, ceasing to cause contraction as smooth movement becomes threatened by overactivation. It is likely that this feedforward mechanism works in concert with others influencing the motoneurons.[5]

Evarts (1973) in summarizing the results of his elegant brain-recording research on the motor system made a statement that expresses one of the main guiding principles of this book. In closing this section, I shall quote from his statement:

> The implications of the studies I have described thus extend into the areas of psychology and psychiatry. Indeed, it seems possible that understanding of the human nervous system, even its most complex intellectual functions, may be enriched if the operation of the brain is analyzed in terms of its motor output rather than in terms of its sensory input. In the past most attempts to describe the higher functions of the brain have been made in terms of how sensory inputs are processed from the receptor on up to the higher cortical centers. A strong case for an alternative approach has been made by Roger W. Sperry of the California Institute of Technology (p. 103).

Sperry's Principle

From an objective, analytical standpoint, Sperry (1952) has stated that it is readily apparent that the sole product of brain function is muscular coordination. Of course he includes neurohumoral and glandular components under motor functions, but he assigns them a relatively minor role in his discussion of the mind-brain problem. Putting the matter in another way, Sperry stated that from his studies of the brain, he believes that the entire output of our thinking mechanism goes into the motor system.

In lower vertebrates, like fish and salamanders, where thought processes are presumably negligible, practically the entire nervous system is clearly concerned with moving the animal about. In the context of Dar-

---

[5] The interested reader may pursue this topic further by referring to Evarts, E. V. V. Feedback and corollary discharge: A merging of the concepts. *Neurosciences Research Program Bulletin*, 1971, *9*, 86–112.

winian evolution theory, it is obvious that the main function of the brain must be that of moving the animal in ways that are advantageous for satisfying basic needs and avoiding dangers.

The important thing we learn from comparative neurology is this: From the fishes to ourselves there is only a gradual elaboration of brain structures, with persistence of the fundamental principles of operation, and always the involvement of the motor system. It is especially significant that Sperry singled out *thought* in placing stress on the unique importance of the motor system; because in eliminating outmoded concepts of thought based on oversimplified motor theories, psychology has apparently gone too far in the opposite direction, so that now the importance of the motor system is in danger of being understated.

As an example of an outmoded concept, some psychologists used to believe that feedback from the tendon receptors in the muscles was required in order to keep the brain active. We now know that brain cells do not require this kind of stimulation to be active. This notion was disproved when electroencephalography showed the brain to be continually active even when the person was immobilized (by anesthesia for instance). Another outmoded idea was that muscle contractions themselves (especially laryngeal ones) *were* thought. This is not at all what Sperry means. His principle states that any directed, organized behavior sequence (including thought) involves the motor system. The muscles are the terminals of this system and, of course, are required for activities like walking, running, and speaking; but the principle, as stated here, does not require that muscles actually have to contract in order for thinking to occur. However, when sensitive electromyography has been used, muscular activity has almost invariably been recorded during thinking (a point that we shall return to presently). Electromyography in these instances shows that the motor system is involved in the "silent acts," because the EMGs reflect what is going on upstream in the brain. On the basis of the available evidence it would be premature to say that the feedforward and feedback loops involving, say, the speech muscles, are completely useless. The point is that the Sperry principle is in no way critically dependent on the presence of *muscle contractions* per se.

FURTHER DATA ON EMG ACCOMPANIMENTS OF THINKING AND RELATED ACTIVITIES

Edmund Jacobson, a great pioneer in this research area, began his career as a psychologist who was interested in a theoretical problem of the 1920s: whether it was possible to engage in thought in the absence of sensations from the muscles. Some psychologists, incidentally, became exceedingly sensitive to sensations from the muscles (including the muscles of speech); and they uniformly reported that their thinking was characteristically accompanied by kinesthetic sensations.[6]

In order to make the methodology in this research more objective, Jacobson in 1927 set about to record muscle tension electrically. With the help of engineers at Bell Telephone Laboratories, Jacobson constructed an electromyograph which, for his purpose, was excellent, and in many respects more satisfactory than ones commercially available, even today. Most important, it was highly sensitive. Jacobson used his electromyograph in an important series of experiments. From the results of these thorough, careful studies, which he conducted at the University of Chicago in the 1920s and 1930s, he was able to conclude with confidence that his fellow psychologists, "the introspectionists," had been correct about the close relation between thinking and muscle tension.

In these studies of muscle tension during thinking, it was necessary to teach the subjects to relax. Because of his training in experiments on introspection of kinesthetic sensations (and the necessity to relax the muscles in these experiments), Jacobson was an expert at relaxing his muscles one by one. He taught this technique, which he called "progressive relaxation," to persons participating in his experiments. With a background of nearly complete relaxation, the slight tensions developing with the onset of thinking were plain to see in the electromyograms. The contractions were generally minute, although sometimes they were grossly visible. In observations involving abstract thought, muscle potentials from the speech musculature were especially conspicuous. Jacobson also reported that his subjects found that they engaged in mental activity less and less as they approached complete relaxation. In addition to being a psychophysiologist, Jacobson is also a physician. In later years, as previously mentioned, he applied his knowledge of muscle tension in treating patients (see Jacobson, 1938, 1970), but he also continued his psychophysiological research. In his laboratory and clinic, Jacobson has improved the sensitivity and reliability of his "integrating neurovoltmeter" from year to year since 1934 and has used it continuously during the decades for measurement of muscle activities during thinking, relaxation, and many "tension states," in health and disease.[7]

[6] For a historical account of this and related work, and for a penetrating analysis of relations between thought and motor action, see Humphrey (1951). For an excellent current review of this research area (including a paper by Edmund Jacobson), see McGuigan and Schoonover (1973).

[7] Jacobson's research had considerable influence on Russian psychologists who have replicated some of his experiments (see Sokolov, 1972). McGuigan (1970) has reviewed that part of Jacobson's research related to McGuigan's interest in EMG recording during reading and other language tasks. McGuigan's review may be consulted for details concerning the experiments of Jacobson and others (including the extensive work of McGuigan himself and his colleagues).

Roland C. Davis was another great pioneer in psychophysiology who investigated thinking.[8] In one set of experiments, Davis (1939) recorded muscle potentials from subjects engaged either in mental multiplication or in memorizing. His results confirmed the earlier findings of Jacobson and others showing that in almost all persons muscular activity was greater during mental work than during rest. Davis' subjects reported a strong tendency to write during mental multiplication. This fits with his finding of higher tension levels in the muscles from the right arm than from the left, in these right-handed subjects. However, the subjects did not say they felt an inclination to write during memorization; and as would be expected from this, no significant difference between left- and right-arm tension was observed in this task.

F. J. McGuigan's extensive EMG research is pursuing these problems and related ones with considerable success. In following up the work of L. W. Max, another pioneer in the EMG-thought research area, McGuigan (1973) studied deaf persons proficient in manual speech, who were learning oral speech. McGuigan found that arm and lip EMGs significantly increased over baseline values during problem solving.

McGuigan has also been conducting research bearing on practical problems related to teaching children to read. The weight of the evidence obtained by McGuigan supports the conclusion that sensitive EMG recording from speech muscles usually reveals more activity during periods of silent reading than during control periods. These results were obtained with adults as well as with children, although the EMGs were higher in children. On the basis of his own research and related work by other investigators, McGuigan believes that teachers are making a mistake when they attempt to eliminate "subvocal" speech during silent reading. He believes that the child needs to subvocalize while reading, and that in time the subvocalization becomes much reduced in the absence of prodding by the teacher.

The fact that the subvocalization becomes reduced seems significant in relation to an earlier warning to the reader: to avoid falling into the trap of believing that *muscular* contractions are essential per se for covert acts like thinking and silent reading. Remember, it is the *motor system* that is indispensable. In learning to read, the child is undoubtedly hindered by the teacher trying to eliminate the visible lip movements too early in the process. In so doing, the teacher is perhaps interfering with the motor system as a whole. Eventually the child learns to reduce (and

---

[8] Roland C. Davis was an observer in our laboratory on the day we recorded EMGs from the hallucinating person, and he concurred in the conclusions that we drew from those observations. Although he did not study EMG gradients extensively, he reported seeing them in his own EMG recording.

later to *nearly* eliminate) the peripheral (muscular) activity, because it is more efficient (and more conventional) to read without it.

McGuigan (1970) is one of the few electromyographers to have recorded from an hallucinating person. In agreement with our findings and those of others reviewed by him, he found that auditory hallucinations were accompanied by EMGs from the speech muscles.

MOTOR THEORIES OF PERCEPTION

The evidence from the EMG research reviewed in the previous sections provides strong support for the proposition that the motor system is an indispensable part of all the activities of the mind. In this section, we briefly review two quite different experimental approaches to perception, which provide additional strong support for this proposition.

Perception of the Speech Code

Liberman, Cooper, Shankweiler, and Studdert-Kennedy (1967) reviewed studies in their laboratory on perception of the speech code. The aim of these studies was to identify the conditions that underlie the perception of speech.

The problem basically was to understand how *phonemes* are perceived. The *phoneme* is "the shortest segment that makes a significant difference between utterances. . . . There are, for example, three such segments in the word 'bad'—/b/, /æ/, and /d/—established by the contrasts with 'dad,' 'bed' and 'bat.' "

In undertaking research to determine how the phoneme is perceived, Liberman and his colleagues considered two very different possibilities: one, a mechanism that operates on a purely auditory basis; the other, by reference to the processes of speech production. Their research supported the latter, which is a *motor* theory. For instance, acoustic patterns for phonemes seen in spectrograms (recordings of the physical characteristics of the spoken sounds) were quite different for the same phonemes from one time to the next, which poses a serious difficulty for the theory of pure auditory decoding. The most parsimonious theory turned out to be one that viewed perception as being mediated by the neural correlates of the motor articulation required to speak the phoneme. Liberman and his colleagues explicitly state that they are talking about the *motor system*, and not about dependence on feedback from muscle contractions and associated muscle receptor discharge.

The Motor System and Visual Perception

Sperry (1952) has stated his principle in relation to perception as follows:

> If there be any objectively demonstrable fact about perception that indicates the nature of the neural process involved, it is the following: In so far as an organism perceives a given object, it is prepared to respond with reference to it. This preparation-to-respond is absent in an organism that has failed to perceive. . . . The presence or absence of adaptive reaction potentialities of this sort, ready to discharge into motor patterns, makes the difference between perceiving and not perceiving (p. 301).

Festinger, Burnham, Ono, and Bamber (1967) reported results of experiments which showed that the visual perceptions of persons in their experiments were influenced by motor actions that they made in relation to the things being perceived.

In one experiment, the person put on some glasses with prisms that made a straight line appear curved. The line was flanked on both sides by brass rods that conducted electricity. The person was given a metal stylus. In one experimental group, the person was told to move the stylus quickly from one end to the other and try to avoid hitting the rods. (Hitting a rod closed an electrical circuit, causing a buzzer to sound.) Since in reality the line was straight (although the prisms made it look curved), in order to avoid hitting the rods the person had to learn to move the arm in a straight line. It turned out that introducing this motor act made the line actually *look* less curved through the prism than in the case of other persons whose motor act was designed to minimize the learning of a new sensory-motor association. This was shown by having persons in both groups turn a knob that controlled a device for putting curvature into a straight line. Persons in both groups were asked to remove their glasses and turn the knob until the curvature of the line matched the curvature of the line that they had been looking at with their glasses on. The group with the training technique designed to *maximize* the learning of a new sensory-motor association produced lines with less curvature than the persons in the other group.[9]

The authors concluded that their results were consistent with a *motor readiness* theory of visual perception of contour. In general, they support Sperry's principle, and once again show the pervasive influence of the motor system.

The reader will recall that in beginning our discussion of EMG

[9] A number of control conditions were used in order to equate the two groups in all respects except for the critical difference in minimizing and maximizing the learning of a new sensory-motor association.

gradients and behavior we stressed the importance of seeing stimuli and responses as inextricably tied together (as two continuously interacting factors in a continuous behavior sequence). It may seem, in our concentration on the response side, that we have seriously neglected the stimulus side. This is surely not intended.

Thinking usually suffers when patterned sensory stimulation is drastically reduced. This fact has been repeatedly demonstrated in experiments, where typically the eyes of reclining subjects are covered with translucent plastic, the hands are enclosed in tubes, and the ears are covered with earphones from which comes constant buzzing. Subjects in a situation of this kind generally complain of being unable to think coherently. These experiments show that, generally speaking, we depend on an adequately stimulating environment for continuous well-organized and effective mental activity (see Zubek, 1969).

Furthermore, Sprague, Chambers, and Stellar (1961) in experiments with cats have demonstrated that sensory deprivation of the forebrain by lesions in the brain stem results in striking behavioral abnormalities.

This discussion anticipates an important principle, which will be dealt with extensively in Chapter VI. This principle states that brain activities converging on the motor system have two main components, one of which is *selective pull* by significant environmental cues, interacting with *push*. (Brain mechanisms for the latter will be discussed in Chapter VI.)

PHENOMENA ASSOCIATED WITH MUSCULAR RELAXATION

Relaxation after Gradient

As we observed earlier, EMG gradients generally reach a peak toward the end of a behavioral sequence, and then characteristically muscle tension falls precipitously when the sequence is completed. This postsequence or posttask relaxation is an interesting phenomenon in its own right.

The rate of the terminal fall also seems to have psychological significance. A prompt, large EMG drop generally coincides with successful completion of a task, giving the person a "feeling of closure." A much slower fall in muscle tension, on the other hand, is usually associated with something not quite complete or not fully satisfying about the performance (or other behavioral sequence). Some examples will clarify the point.

Early in our series of experiments on the physiological gradient phenomenon, Smith (1953) found that muscle tension (EMG) dropped significantly more after completion than after interruption of our mirror drawing task. This fits nicely with Kurt Lewin's theory, according to which task interruption serves to continue or prolong a "tension system." For

discussion of Lewin's theory (with particular reference to task completion) in relation to a similar theoretical approach, see Miller, Galanter,
and Pribram's (1960) book, and see also Malmo (1965).

EMGs in Interpersonal Interaction

Drop in muscle tension at the conclusion of an interpersonal exchange can be observed under controlled laboratory conditions. We
recorded from interacting pairs, first from a patient and examining psychologist, and immediately afterwards (as explained below) from the
same patient and a psychiatrist. Nineteen patients participated in the
experiment: nine in the praised group and ten in the criticized group.
When the psychologist *praised* the patients for good performance on a
test (telling a story about a picture), their speech-muscle tension fell
sharply—and so did the speech-muscle tension of the psychologist! But
when the psychologist *criticized* the patient's story, the patient's speech-
muscle tension did not fall (nor did the psychologist's). In other words,
after criticism, there was "residual tension." Our EMGs showed that the
patient's residual tension could be removed through reassurance afterwards by another member of the research team (see Malmo, Boag, &
Smith, 1957).

Muscular Relaxation Produced by Curare-Type Drugs

As stated earlier, the presence of *muscle contraction* per se is not
regarded as critical for demonstrating the unique importance of the motor
system for psychology. However, it is of some interest to examine the
findings obtained in experiments where muscle contractions have been
eliminated (or nearly so) by means of pharmacological blockades (for
example, curare drugs), which interfere with the stimulation of muscle
fibers by their motoneurons.

Hodes (1962) found that when he injected Flaxedil (a curare drug)
into the veins of cats, they became sleepy, and their EEGs changed from
a desynchronized pattern characteristic of an alert state, to a synchronized pattern characteristic of a less alert state. (See again Figure 3.9
and accompanying text.)

Hodes proved that the Flaxedil was in fact producing its effect through
blocking muscle activity. When he injected the drug into the brain directly
through the carotid artery, which is the direct supply route for blood to
the brain, the effect was not produced. This means that the Flaxedil was
ineffective in blocking the transmission from the axonal terminals of
neurons to the cell body on which they converged. These junctions between
neurons, called *synapses* evidently are relatively unaffected by curare-type

drugs. Curare drugs (like Flaxedil) do block the transmission from the motoneurons to the muscle fiber. This junction is called the *myoneural junction*. There is evidently something about the biochemical events taking place during transmission through this junction that makes it particularly vulnerable to being blocked by curare.

In interpreting his results, Hodes stressed the probable importance of a feedback system originating in the muscle receptors, and involving circuitous pathways in the cerebellum with inputs to the cerebral cortex. The cerebellum is the structure, with many thin convolutions, at the rear of the brain. It is known that impulses from muscle and tendon receptors are carried in the spinal columns directly to the cerebellum. The cerebellum also has an important input into the reticular core, which will be discussed in Chapter V (see Figure 5.3). Hodes' experiment will be considered again in Chapter V.

These experimental findings of Hodes should caution us against concluding prematurely that muscular contractions per se are unimportant for normal functioning of the brain.

Because curare paralyzes muscles for breathing, animals must be artificially respired when injected with the drug. Considering the hazards involved, it is understandable that people do not wish to be injected with curare, in order to report on its effects. To the best of my knowledge, there is only one published account of an investigation in which a person was injected with a curare drug and then observed for as long as a half hour. As the following account states, soon after injection with the curare drug (d-tubocurarine) the subject reported that he found it difficult "to focus on anything." This suggests an interference with thinking, which unfortunately was not adequately tested in this experiment. However, as the following description indicates, the man retained consciousness.

Curare Injections in a Man   Because curare is useful in some surgical operations, anesthesiologists have long been interested in the effects of curare on the nervous system. Smith, Brown, Toman, and Goodman (1947) administered curare (d-tubocurarine) to a healthy male subject with the purpose of determining the "cerebral effects" of curare. The log commenced at 2:00 P.M. and continued until 6:00 P.M. At 2:11 P.M. d-tubocurarine chloride was injected intravenously at a slow constant rate over a period of 15 minutes. The subject reported feeling "a little bit dizzy and quite a 'glow.'" He found it "a little hard to focus on anything." He reported weakness in his jaw muscles, that it was difficult to talk, to swallow, and to keep his eyes open, and he said that his legs felt weak. He said that he felt "no unpleasant sensations." At 2:18, at the subject's request, artificial respiration commenced. At 2:20 speech was no longer possible, but he could hear distinctly and was able to nod his head and to move his hands slightly, although he could scarcely move his fingers.

Gradually the subject lost control of limb muscles, neck muscles, and forehead muscles (in that order apparently). When all other muscle control had disappeared, the subject still retained slight movement of his left eyebrow. This was the last remaining means of communication with the investigators. At 2:42 P.M. the left-eyebrow movement was very slight, but he was still able to use it to signal in answer to inquiries that his sensations were intact, and that he could feel painful stimuli. He also indicated that he wished to be injected with more d-tubocurarine chloride. (Since the first injection, he had been injected twice more at his request by signaling with his left eyebrow.)

At 2:45 P.M. the subject was unable to signal response to inquiries, due to complete skeletal muscular paralysis. The subject was in this completely paralyzed state for six minutes. At 2:51 P.M. neostigmine methylsulfate, a substance that counteracts the effects of curare, was administered intravenously. By 2:56 P.M. the subject was able to contract the left eyebrow muscles again. The remainder of the log described the return of muscular control as more and more neostigmine methylsulfate was administered.

From their observations, the investigators concluded that "at no time was there any evidence of lapse of consciousness." They also interpreted the EEG as being normal throughout the period of paralysis. However, they realized afterwards that they should have attempted to arrange some means of communication during the period of complete muscular paralysis. One of the procedures they thought might have worked was recording action potentials from the end-plate region of the muscle that the subject was attempting to contract. Besides missing this opportunity it was also unfortunate that the procedures of mental testing that they used were not described in greater detail. From the rather sketchy account, their mental tests appeared easy.

Despite these shortcomings, their investigation does appear to demonstrate that a man can remain conscious even though paralyzed by curare to the point where he cannot signal with any muscle. The subject stated afterwards that he was entirely conscious during the period of complete muscular paralysis, and he showed by objective tests of recall that he had memory for events during this period. Again, it is unfortunate that EMGs were not recorded, not only as a possible means for the subject to signal, but in order to test the limits of skeletal-muscle paralysis, because as the reader will recall, our EMG gradients were generally recorded from muscles that were *not* involved in visible movement either.

To repeat, it is of particular interest that the subject said he found it difficult to focus on anything. This suggests impairment of thought processes, and again it is unfortunate that the subject's thinking abilities under

the drug were not more adequately assessed. There is a tremendous difference between simply being conscious versus engaging in high-level psychological activities (such as problem solving and the like). Until these
capacities *are* tested under curare, the *possibility* of muscle contractions
being important for certain psychological activities must be respected;
although as has been pointed out repeatedly, the question of functional
participation of *muscle contractions* per se in psychological functions is
not a critical one for the principle that we have been discussing.

DISTINCTIVE FEATURES OF THE HUMAN BRAIN

In this chapter we have examined a substantial amount of evidence
supporting the Sperry principle. This evidence, which was drawn from a
great variety of sources, has supported the principle which states that the
motor system is indispensable for all psychological functions.

The motor system is comprised of various brain areas that project
directly to the final common pathway where they converge on motoneurons
in the ventral horn of the spinal cord (and in the motor nuclei of the
cranial nerves). The principle is applicable to animals from fishes to man.
The fact that the operation of man's brain follows this general principle
stresses the similarities between human and infrahuman animals. However,
there are tremendous differences between ourselves and the monkeys and
apes. Probably the most conspicuous difference is our capacity for complex language. Therefore, it should be worthwhile to compare the brains
of human and infrahuman primates in order to see what we can make of
the differences that have been found in investigations to date.

Man's neocortex (the outer layer of the brain) is roughly three times
as large as one would expect in a primate with the same size of body
(Passingham, 1973). This probably accounts in large part for our brain's
greater capacity for what D. O. Hebb calls "holding" ("the capacity of
the brain to receive an excitation and transmit it to muscle or gland after
some appreciable period of time").

In most respects man's neocortex is quite similar to that of the
monkeys and apes, and where there are differences, generally they are
merely related to the differences in total size of the neocortex. However,
Geschwind and Levitsky's (1968) study of 100 human brains suggests
that there may be a difference in one neocortical area, representing a
significant exception to the general rule. This area, which is in the left
temporal lobe, is known to be important for finding the right words when
speaking. It is called Wernicke's area, named for the man who first
described this form of difficulty with speech. In Wernicke's aphasia the
patient fails to use the correct word and substitutes circumlocutory phrases
("what you use to write with" for "pencil") and words without specific

meaning ("thing," "the other one"). In 65 percent of the normal brains studied, this area was larger on the left than on the right side; while it was larger on the right in only 11 percent of the cases. It is generally supposed that comparable differences between right and left sides are absent in infrahuman primates, although precise measurement must be done in order to establish the point.

In Broca's aphasia, named after Paul Broca, who in 1861 published the first of a series of papers on language and the brain, the patient has great difficulty getting out any words at all. His speech is slow and labored, and his articulation is crude. This kind of aphasia is associated with damage to a brain area that lies forward in the brain from Wernicke's area, and it is almost invariably on the left side. Neurosurgeons Penfield and Roberts (1959) have summarized their extensive observations of the effects of electrically stimulating Broca's area in conscious patients during brain operations, which were carried out under local anesthesia (because cutting brain tissue is painless). Stimulation of Broca's area elicits vocalization that takes the form of a sustained or interrupted vowel cry, which at times may have a consonant component. No intelligible word was ever elicited by electrical brain stimulation. Organized speech cannot be elicited by brain stimulation because speech depends on sequential ordering (which means the sequential firing of a chain of neurons in a certain order over a period of time). Brain stimulation, which fires all the neurons in the chain at the same time, interferes with the ordered sequence so that all that comes out is a cry. As a matter of fact, if the patient happens to be speaking when the stimulation comes on, this organized speech ceases for the entire period of stimulation. The purpose of these stimulations during operation is to enable the brain surgeon to identify areas essential for vocalization and speech, so that he can avoid damage to them.

Electrical stimulation of the homologous neocortical area in the squirrel monkey by Jürgens and Ploog (1970) failed to produce any vocalization, although many *sub*cortical areas did produce vocalization when stimulated. Their report was based on stimulating at 5940 electrode sites in thirty-nine squirrel monkeys, who are good subjects for this kind of study because they possess a rich vocal repertoire made up of easily distinguishable vocalization types. According to students of squirrel monkey behavior, the different vocalizations are related to distinct behaviors: for example, growling has been interpreted as an expression of directed aggressiveness (occurring in connection with specific dominance gestures). "Quacking" is a typical call of irritation, and expresses a state ranging between uneasiness and threatening behavior. "Shrieking" represents the highest degree of excitement.

These calls elicited by brain stimulation sounded like the calls that the monkeys made in their cages. However, there appeared to be a significant difference between the way they were elicited from the monkeys and the way the vowel sounds were elicited from the human patients. In the case of the patients, the electrode appeared to be placed directly in a neocortical motor speech area, whereas in the case of the monkeys, as previously mentioned, stimulation of their neocortical homologues failed to produce any vocalization at all. In the monkeys, the sites producing vocalization were of two general kinds. One was in or very close to a subcortical *motor system* in the midbrain and the other (with longer latencies: that is, taking longer for the stimulation to produce its effect) was *not* in a motor system at all, but in what is called the *limbic system*. This is extremely interesting because the monkey calls have strong emotional significance, and the limbic system is considered to play a key role in emotional behavior. Robinson (1967) who had conducted a similar detailed investigation, using rhesus monkeys, concluded as follows: "Primate vocalization is used principally as threat, aggression, fear, pain, pleasure, feeding, and separation." Limbic means "forming a ring or border." As will be noted in Figure 3.16, the several structures in the schematic represenation of the limbic system have the appearance of a ring; and it was Broca who introduced the term *limbic lobe* in referring to the upper ring. Limbic structures include parts of the brain previously thought to be chiefly involved in the sense of smell, and for this reason they were previously referred to as *olfactory brain* or *rhinencephalon*. Because many limbic structures are involved in the functioning of the autonomic nervous system, these structures have also been called the *visceral brain*. In 1937 Papez (pronounced "papes") published a paper that was prescient. He called attention to part of what is now referred to as the limbic system as forming a circuit that he thought would turn out to be important in relation to emotions. In the current literature one sometimes sees references to the "Papez circuit." The term limbic system was coined by MacLean, whose writings will be discussed in Chapter VII.

Most limbic structures have an intermediate position in the brain, and their significance for behavior must therefore be reckoned in relation to their influence via their projections to the midbrain and the reticular core. The relations of the hypothalamus and other limbic structures with the midbrain are described in Chapter V (see Figure 5.3 and the accompanying text). In short, as Pribram and Kruger (1954) have indicated in their classical paper, the limbic system is an integral part of the whole brain. The structures of the limbic system may be viewed as playing an intermediating role in relaying neural impulses to the midbrain, there to connect with neurons that are part of the motor system, and thence to the muscles (and to their supporting physiological mechanisms) for action.

The balance of evidence favors the conclusion that some of our own deplorable conduct, for example, acts of hostile aggression, pushing over others in panic situations, and the like, strongly involve the limbic system, that is, the homologues of the limbic structures, which have been extensively studied in animals. Actually, there are clinical data to support this conclusion (MacLean, 1964).

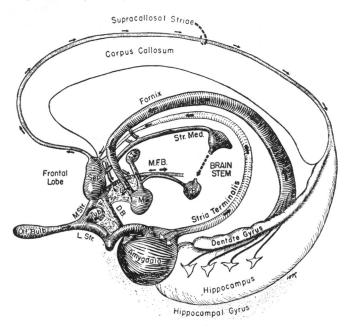

Figure 3.16. *Diagram showing parts of the limbic system.* Fornix forms outer part of the upper ring and hippocampus outer part of the lower ring. See Figure 5.3 and the accompanying text for a description of the brain stem and its relations with the hypothalamus and other limbic structures. Some of the limbic structures that Jürgens and Ploog (1970) found to be involved in the different vocalizations in their squirrel monkeys were as follows: cackling calls: amygdala; growling calls: posterior hypothalamus, stria terminalis, and amygdala; trilling: fornix; chirping: hippocampus; shrieking: stria terminalis and hypothalamus. Abbreviations: A. T., anterior nucleus of thalamus; D. B., diagonal band of Broca; H., habenula; I. P., interpeduncular nucleus; L. Str., lateral olfactory stria; M., mammillary body (a part of the posterior hypothalamus); M. F. B., medial forebrain bundle; M. Str., medial olfactory stria; Olf. Bulb, olfactory bulb; Sep., region of the septal nuclei; Str. Med., stria medullaris; Tub., olfactory tubercle. (From MacLean, Psychosomatic disease and the "visceral brain." *Psychosomatic Medicine*, 1949, *11*, 338–353.)

In order for animals to survive in the wilds, they require specialized brain mechanisms that enable them to cope with emergencies, where they must fight or flee. In Chapter V we discuss how these same mechanisms operative in our own civilized society can be extremely disadvantageous for us. Here then are some of the reasons why we must view our brains as archaic, that is, more appropriate for an earlier, more primitive time than for modern social living.

A word should be said about the kind of evolutionary process that most likely has produced our brains. In lecturing on evolution of the brain, W. Nauta employs a simile that illustrates a point of key significance. In building a new highway, an entirely new surface is laid down. An old dirt road that the new highway replaces is either bypassed or else paved over completely. It would be considered stupid to add only a thin strip of paving along the entire length of the dirt road so that no more than two wheels of an automobile could roll over the new portion, while the other two wheels bumped along over the old rough road. Yet the brain has evolved in just such an ill-planned manner. Most of the structures in our brain can be easily traced all through the animal series down to the fishes, and the changes are makeshift "add-ons" in the nature of Nauta's simile about the roads.

Suppose we return to the difference between human speech and monkey vocalization. On the basis of the preceding neuroanatomical discussion, we are able to see the possibility of quite an important difference between the two.

It is possible, it seems, for the neurosurgeon to stimulate Broca's area in a patient, and to produce vocalization without involving the limbic system. There are motor pathways that go directly from Broca's area to the speech muscles. On the other hand, the data from related monkey experiments clearly suggest that it is impossible to produce vocalization without the limbic system.

If further research bears this out, it would unquestionably represent the most radical known neuroanatomical difference between monkey and man. As Robinson has suggested, if this is the case then the neocortical structures mediating human speech have a distinct advantage in their relative detachment from brain mechanisms concerned with primitive functions such as fighting, running, eating, drinking, and sexual activity, in addition to advantages accruing from structures providing for vastly increased information-carrying capacity, as evidenced in human speech and in written language.

Despite this advance, however, our brains still retain many archaic features. Referring again to Nauta's simile, this apparent advance in the human brain is like that thin strip of paved road. The detachment of the neural mechanism for speech *is* only relative. Broca's area has neural connections with the prefrontal lobes, which are situated just in front of it. The prefrontal lobes project in turn directly to the hypothalamus (being the only neocortical area to do so), and Nauta regards the prefrontal lobes themselves as part of the limbic system. Furthermore, Broca's area and other brain areas serving language functions are potentially under the influence of subcortical structures through fiber tracts ascending from the reticular core (see Chapter V) as well as through other channels.

Finally, speech and language functions are generally part of an extensive activation of the entire motor system.

Most persons would be inclined to believe that certain highly superior individuals (like Einstein) must be free from the handicaps that we have been talking about in connection with archaic features of the human brain. Einstein was in the habit of saying that he wrote about *objective* matters. No doubt his theoretical thinking (and that of most physicists and mathematicians) was exceedingly objective. Yet even Einstein was almost emotional in his attacks on quantum theory. Einstein wrote to one of its proponents, "In our scientific expectation we have become antipodes. You believe in God playing dice and I in perfect laws in the world of things existing as real objects, which I try to grasp in a wildly speculative way."

Actually, Einstein, in dealings with people with whom he had scientific differences, demonstrated a sense of mutual respect, and everyone was impressed with his benevolence. Newton was vastly different. Newton waged savage personal warfare against all his contemporaries who had ideas of their own. He was subject to vicious rages in demolishing anyone he regarded as a rival.

In conclusion, we seem to have a glimpse of a significant advance in "brain design" in going from monkeys to ourselves. But at the same time we can perhaps perceive the archaic aspects of our brain a little more clearly, and realize that some of these archaic features and their unfortunate consequences are inherent in the evolutionary process.

SUMMARY

Slow, steadily progressive rise in forehead muscle tension was monitored electromyographically in a frontal headache patient during a stressful interview. When the muscle tension had climbed to a high point, the patient complained of frontal headache. This observation represents a specific instance of an extremely pervasive phenomenon, which we call the *electromyographic (EMG) gradient*.

EMG gradients appear only in certain muscles. Persons with complaints of discomfort from excessive muscle tension are more inclined to show EMG gradients in the troublesome muscle group than in other muscle groups. However, EMG gradients are observed in recordings from nearly all persons, not just from those with complaints of overtense muscles.

There are also situational differences. For example, during tracking with the right arm, EMG gradients are usually prominent in recordings from the nontracking left forearm muscles, whereas listening attentively to a story usually results in EMG gradients appearing in recordings from the forehead muscles.

Steepness of the gradient is a significant feature. Generally speaking, the stronger the person's involvement in what he or she is doing, the steeper the gradient. EMG gradients usually fail to appear with psychologically low-level repetitive types of activity (for example, simple tapping on a telegraph key).

EMG gradients have been observed in decision making and in various other kinds of goal-directed behavior. Gradients have been observed in EMG recording during various silent, muted activities (even in hallucinations).

The pervasiveness of EMG gradients is one of several lines of evidence that support Sperry's principle. According to this principle, the entire output of our thinking mechanism goes into the motor system. From the fishes to ourselves there is only a gradual elaboration of brain structures, with persistence of the fundamental principles of operation, and always the involvement of the motor system. However, the principle does *not* require that muscles actually contract in order for thinking to take place.

The motor system is highly complex, involving a large number of structures, all capable of influencing muscle contractions. There are two kinds of muscle fiber. *Ordinary* muscle fibers are designed to move a bony lever when the fibers contract. A second kind of muscle fiber (*modified* or *intrafusal* muscle fiber) also contracts (shortens) except for its central part, which contains sensory endings. These sensory endings are stimulated when the intrafusal fiber contracts. Sensory fibers go from the sensory endings to the spinal cord and, by means of connections to higher brain centers, serve in feedback loops for purposes of motor coordination. Unlike ordinary muscle fibers, intrafusal muscle fibers do not pull on a bony lever.

It appears from the experimental evidence that sometimes, at least, EMG gradients may be largely a function of activated intrafusal muscle fibers. Having their own motor nerve fibers, the intrafusal fibers can be activated while the ordinary muscle fibers remain inactive.

The nerve fiber that activates the muscle fiber is called the *motoneuron*, and its cell body lies in the ventral horn of the spinal cord. There is a convergence on the motoneuron from some seven or more different brain areas. The motor system is comprised of brain structures that project *directly* to the motoneurons in the ventral horns of the spinal cord (and to the motor nuclei of the cranial nerves).

Evidence from the EMG research reviewed in this chapter provides strong support for the proposition that the motor system is an indispensable part of all the activities of the mind. Additional support for this proposition was noted in connection with the research by Liberman and his colleagues on perception of the speech code. In undertaking research to determine how speech is perceived, they considered two very different possibilities: one, a mechanism that operates on a purely auditory basis; the other, by reference to the processes of speech production. Their research supported the latter, which is a *motor theory*. The most parsimonious theory turned out to be one that viewed perception of speech as being mediated by the neural correlates of the motor articulation required to speak the *phoneme* (the shortest speech segment that makes a significant difference between utterances).

Further support for Sperry's principle as applied to perception was noted in the research on visual perception by Festinger and his colleagues, who showed that the visual perceptions of persons in their experiments were influenced by motor actions that they made in relation to the things being perceived.

When we turned from considering motor system activation to considering phenomena of muscular relaxation, we noted a number of interesting points. EMG gradients generally reach a peak toward the end of a behavioral sequence, and then, when the sequence is completed, tension falls precipitously. The rate of terminal fall seems to have psychological significance. A prompt, large EMG drop generally coincides with successful completion of a task, giving the person a "feeling of closure." A much slower fall in muscle tension, on the other hand, is usually associated with something not quite complete or not fully satisfying about the performance (or other behavioral sequence).

There are individual differences in the ability to relax, and persons who find it extremely difficult to relax (like the chronic anxiety patients described in the previous chapter) benefit from special treatments designed to produce muscular relaxation. Jacobson's "progressive relaxation" technique is one example of such a treatment.

Jacobson also reported that his subjects found that they engaged in mental activity less and less as they approached complete relaxation. R. C. Davis confirmed these earlier findings of Jacobson and others, showing that in almost all persons muscular activity was greater during mental work than during rest.

Finally, we considered the question whether there are features of the human brain that represent a radical departure from the brains of lower primates. In a study of 100 human brains, Geschwind and Levitsky found an area in the left temporal lobe (Wernicke's speech area) which in 65 percent of the brains was larger on the left than on the right side. On the right side it was larger in only 11 percent of the cases. It is generally supposed that comparable differences between right and left sides are absent in infrahuman primates, although precise measurements must be done in order to establish this point.

Observations of the effects of brain stimulation on vocalization in conscious patients (under local anesthesia) and in infrahuman primates suggest the intriguing possibility that whereas the brain areas mediating monkeys' vocalizations are confined to structures outside the neocortex, human vocalization (and speech) are mediated chiefly by the neocortex.

Limbic system structures were especially prominent among those that produced monkey vocalizations when stimulated electrically. This is of considerable interest because the monkey calls (which were reproduced by brain stimulation) have strong emotional significance (related to threat, aggression, fear, pain, feeding, and the like). These observations fit well with the widely held view that certain limbic system structures are of key importance for emotional aspects of behavior in all mammals.

If further research confirms this apparent difference between human and infrahuman brains in relation to vocalization, then, as Robinson has suggested, the neocortical structures mediating human speech would be distinctly advantageous in their relative detachment from brain mechanisms concerned with primitive functions such as fighting, running, eating, drinking, and sexual activity, as well as being advantageous in providing for vastly increased information-carrying capacity, as evidenced in human speech and written language.

However radical the neuroanatomical alteration may turn out to be, it is clear from neurophysiological considerations that the detachment of the neural mechanisms for speech and language functions from limbic system structures must be incomplete. Therefore, despite the apparent significant advance, from monkey to man, it seems certain that the human brain is bound to retain archaic features.

In this chapter we have focused on the motor system and the skeletal musculature. In the next chapter the focus will be on the *autonomic* nervous system, which gets its name from the fact that many of its functions operate without our having to attend to them. Actually, the chief role of these autonomic functions may be considered as supporting the activities of the skeletal-motor system.

REFERENCES

Aserinsky, E., & Kleitman, N. Regularly occurring periods of eye motility, and concomitant phenomena, during sleep. *Science*, 1953, *118*, 273–274.

Bartoshuk, A. K. EMG gradients and EEG amplitude during motivated listening. *Canadian Journal of Psychology*, 1956, *10*, 156–164.

Bélanger, D. "Gradients" musculaires et processus mentaux superieurs. *Canadian Journal of Psychology*, 1957, *11*, 113–122.

Davis, F. H., & Malmo, R. B. Electromyographic recording during interview. *American Journal of Psychiatry*, 1951, *107*, 908–916.

Davis, R. C. Patterns of muscular activity during "mental work" and their constancy. *Journal of Experimental Psychology*, 1939, *24*, 451–465.

Edmeads, J. The management of patients with headache. *Therapeutics*, 1971, *1*, 32–39.

Evarts, E. V. *V*. Feedback and corollary discharge: A merging of the concepts. *Neurosciences Research Program Bulletin*, 1971, *9*, 86–112.

Evarts, E. V. Brain mechanisms in movement. *Scientific American*, 1973, *229* (1), 95–103.

Festinger, L., Burnham, C. A., Ono, H., & Bamber, D. Efference and the conscious experience of perception. *Journal of Experimental Psychology Monograph*, 1967, *74*(4, Whole No. 637).

Geschwind, N., & Levitsky, W. Human brain: Left-right asymmetries in temporal speech region. *Science*, 1968, *161*, 186–187.

Hebb, D. O. Discussion of Malmo, R. B. & Bélanger, D. Related physiological and behavioral changes: What are their determinants? In S. Kety, E. V. Evarts, & H. L. Williams (Eds.), *Sleep and altered states of consciousness*. Baltimore: Williams & Wilkins, 1967. P. 315.

Hodes, R. Electrocortical synchronization resulting from reduced proprioceptive drive caused by neuromuscular blocking agents. *Electroencephalography and Clinical Neurophysiology*, 1962, *14*, 220–232.

Humphrey, G. *Thinking. An introduction to its experimental psychology*. New York: Wiley, 1951.

Jacobson, E. *Progressive relaxation*. (2nd ed.) Chicago: University of Chicago Press, 1938.

Jacobson, E. *Modern treatment of tense patients*. Springfield, Ill.: Charles C Thomas, 1970.

Jürgens, U., & Ploog, D. Cerebral representation of vocalization in the squirrel monkey. *Experimental Brain Research*, 1970, *10*, 532–554.

Lang, J. The other side of hallucinations. Part II. Interpretation. *American Journal of Psychiatry*, 1939, *96*, 423–430.

Liberman, A. M., Cooper, F. S., Shankweiler, D. P., & Studdert-Kennedy, M. Perception of the speech code. *Psychological Review*, 1967, *74*, 431–461.

MacLean, P. D. Psychosomatic disease and the "visceral brain." *Psychosomatic Medicine*, 1949, *11*, 338–353.

MacLean, P. D. The limbic system ("visceral brain") in relation to central gray and reticulum of the brain stem. *Psychosomatic Medicine*, 1955, *17*, 355–366.

MacLean, P. D. Man and his animal brains. *Modern Medicine*, 1964, February 3, 95–106.

Malmo, R. B. Activation: A neuropsychological dimension. *Psychological Review*, 1959, *66*, 367–386.

Malmo, R. B. Physiological gradients and behavior. *Psychological Bulletin*, 1965, *64*, 225–234.

Malmo, R. B., Boag, T. J., & Smith, A. A. Physiological study of personal interaction. *Psychosomatic Medicine*, 1957, *19*, 105–119.

Malmo, R. B., & Surwillo, W. W. Sleep deprivation: Changes in performance and physiological indicants of activation. *Psychological Monographs*, 1960, *74*, (Whole No. 502), 1–24.

McGuigan, F. J. Covert oral behavior during the silent performance of language tasks. *Psychological Bulletin*, 1970, *74*, 309–326.

McGuigan, F. J. Electrical measurement of covert processes as an explication of "higher mental events." In F. J. McGuigan & R. A. Schoonover (Eds.), *The psychophysiology of thinking. Studies of covert processes.* New York: Academic Press, 1973. Pp. 343–385.

McGuigan, F. J., & Tanner, R. G. Covert oral behavior during conversational and visual dreams. *Psychonomic Science*, 1971, *23*, 263–264.

Melzack, R. *The puzzle of pain.* Harmondsworth, England: Penguin, 1973.

Merton, P. A. How we control the contraction of our muscles. *Scientific American*, 1972, *226*, 30–37.

Miller, G. A., Galanter, E., & Pribram, K. H. *Plans and the structure of behavior.* New York: Holt, Rinehart and Winston, 1960.

Milner, P. M. *Physiological psychology.* New York: Holt, Rinehart and Winston, 1970.

Passingham, R. E. Anatomical differences between the neocortex of man and other primates. *Brain, Behavior and Evolution*, 1973, *7*, 337–359.

Penfield, W., & Roberts, L. *Speech and brain-mechanisms.* Princeton, New Jersey: Princeton University Press, 1959.

Pribram, K. H. *Languages of the brain: Experimental paradoxes and principles in neuropsychology.* Englewood Cliffs, N.J.: Prentice-Hall, 1971.

Pribram, K. H., & Kruger, L. Functions of the "olfactory brain." *Annals of the New York Academy of Sciences*, 1954, *58*, 109–138.

Robinson, B. W. Vocalization evoked from forebrain in *Macaca mulatta*. *Physiology and Behavior*, 1967, *2*, 345–354.

Shagass, C., & Malmo, R. B. Psychodynamic themes and localized muscular tension during psychotherapy. *Psychosomatic Medicine*, 1954, *16*, 295–313.

Smith, A. A. An electromyographic study of tension in interrupted and completed tasks. *Journal of Experimental Psychology*, 1953, *46*, 32–36.

Smith, S. M., Brown, H. O., Toman, J. E. P., & Goodman, L. S. The lack of cerebral effects of *d*-tubocurarine. *Anesthesiology*, 1947, *8*, 1–14.

Sokolov, A. N. *Inner speech and thought.* (Trans. by G. T. Onischenko) New York: Plenum Press, 1972.

Sperry, R. W. Neurology and the mind-brain problem. *American Scientist*, 1952, *40*, 291–312.

Sprague, J. M., Chambers, W. W., & Stellar, E. Attentive, affective, and adaptive behavior in the cat. *Science*, 1961, *133*, 165–173.

Wallerstein, H. An electromyographic study of attentive listening. *Canadian Journal of Psychology*, 1954, *8*, 228–238.

Weiner, H. Schizophrenia. III: Etiology. In A. M. Freedman & H. I. Kaplan

(Eds.), *Comprehensive textbook of psychiatry*. Baltimore: Williams & Wilkins, 1967. Pp. 603–621.

Zubek, J. P. Sensory and perceptual-motor effects. In J. P. Zubek (Ed.), *Sensory deprivation: Fifteen years of research*. New York: Appleton-Century-Crofts, 1969. Pp. 207–253.

IV

Cold Hands and Other Autonomic Reactions

LILI,[1] A PRETTY TEEN-AGER, suffered from continually cold hands. She was referred to specialists who were making a study of patients with this complaint.

Lili was an only child whose parents separated when she was one year old. At the time of this investigation, she was living with her mother, to whom she was "emotionally attached." However, she was often on bad terms with her mother because of criticisms and disagreements. Since the age of 14 Lili had been a party to numerous sex episodes. She was impulsive and headstrong; her moods changed quickly; and she was easily angered. At times she would not speak to her mother for weeks. Yet she was in conflict because of the emotional attachment to her mother, and resentful because of the dependency.

---

[1] "Lili" is a fictitious name, as are all the other names in the case histories. Lili was a patient investigated in the laboratory by Mittelmann and Wolff (1939), pioneers in this field. Readers interested in further details concerning case histories may consult the original sources.

TEMPERATURE OF HANDS RECORDED DURING MEMORY TEST AND DURING INTERVIEW

In the recording room, Lili rested comfortably on a cushioned examining table. Her hands were placed on a pillow with the fingers close to a radiometer (a sensitive temperature-measuring instrument). Lili was asked to remember, and then to repeat forward and backward, a series of numbers read to her. This test caused the skin temperature of her fingers to drop. Lili considered the procedure a test of her intelligence and was disturbed over mistakes. During rest following this test, after some fluctuations, the temperature of Lili's fingers returned to pretest level.

The doctor then talked to Lili about her mother, with whom she was on bad terms at the time. Skin temperature of the fingers dropped nearly three times as much as it had during the memory test (see Figure 4.1A).

PHYSIOLOGICAL MECHANISMS

Cooling of the hands is due to constriction (narrowing in diameter) of blood vessels in the skin. The mechanisms responsible for this *vasoconstriction* are explained in Figures 4.1B, 4.1C, and 4.1D. Anger, the behavioral reaction illustrated in Figure 4.1D, is integrated by means of a cortical-hypothalamic-midbrain mechanism. The figure is based on numerous animal experiments by neurophysiologists. During electrical stimulation of a cat's hypothalamus near the midline, the cat, with arched back and erect hair, will spit and hiss, and will spring viciously at anyone coming too close.[2]

Hypothalamic stimulation that produces this noisy attack causes constriction of blood vessels in the skin while simultaneously causing dilation of blood vessels in the muscles (see Uvnäs, 1960). Depending on the kind of pattern of neural impulses in the cortical-hypothalamic-midbrain pathways, the behavior may take the form of an angry attack or it may take the form of an emergency reaction. Both utilize physiological mechanisms that prepare the individual for strong muscular exertion (see Uvnäs, 1960). In these situations the constriction of blood vessels in the skin, by giving up blood at the surface, serves the useful purpose of making more blood available to the muscles for strong or violent activity. In the process, of course, the hands become colder.

Constriction of the blood vessels (*vasoconstriction*) in the hands is also part of a heat-conserving mechanism of the body. This mechanism

[2] For discussion of related behaviors produced by other nearby stimulation points in the hypothalamus, see Milner, 1970.

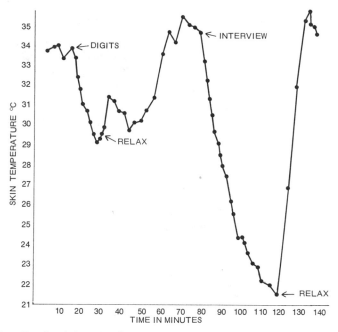

Figure 4.1A *Graph of drop in skin temperature.* Lili's hands become cold during emotion-provoking experiences. Graph shows drops in skin temperature of fingers during memory test and during interview. Lili was worried about her performance on the test. The topic of the interview stirred her to feelings of anger and resentment against her mother. Drops in skin temperature are caused by vasoconstriction, that is, narrowing of the lumens (spaces inside) of the blood vessels. When the diameter of the blood vessels in the skin is reduced (that is, *constricted*), heat loss from the skin is decreased, and radiometer (sensitive temperature-measuring instrument) registers a drop in temperature. The smaller the diameter of the blood vessels in the skin, the smaller the area of warm blood at the surface of the body, and consequently the lower the reading on the radiometer (which measures heat radiating from the body). When the patient relaxes, skin temperature rises. (After Mittelmann & Wolff, Affective states and skin temperature: Experimental study of subjects with "cold hands" and Raynaud's syndrome. *Psychosomatic Medicine,* 1939, *1,* 271–292.)

involves hypothalamic structures different from those serving the preparation for action.

   Suppose we work our way from the *smooth* muscles, which produce the vasoconstriction, up through the spinal cord to the brain. This will give us an opportunity to compare the neural pathways for a *smooth-muscle* (or autonomic) response (see Figure 4.1B) with that for a *skeletal-muscle* (or "optional" or "voluntary") response (refer back to Chapter III).

   Figure 4.1C illustrates a difference between autonomic and skeletal mechanisms at the level of the spinal cord. Whereas the *skeletal* muscle fiber is activated by a motoneuron whose cell body lies within the spinal

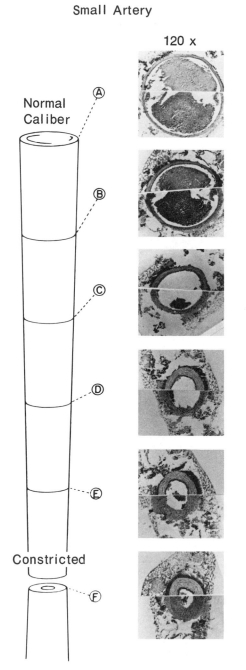

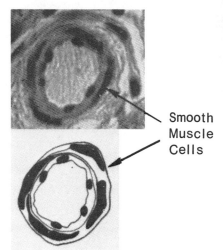

Small Artery

120 x

Terminal Artery

Normal Caliber

Constricted

Smooth Muscle Cells

cord, as is shown in Figure 3.15, the smooth muscle fiber is activated by a *postganglionic* neuron, which is itself activated by a *motoneuron* lying in the lateral horn of the spinal cord. Upstream from this point, the pathways for autonomic smooth-muscle innervation have much in common with those for skeletal-muscle innervation. While it is true that the limbic system (and especially the hypothalamus) is more prominent in autonomic functions, the hypothalamus does not project directly to the autonomic motoneurons in the lateral horns of the spinal cord. As in the case of all limbic-system structures, projection is from the hypothalamus to the midbrain. Downstream from the midbrain, there are some important autonomic centers in the *medulla oblongata* (see Figure 4.1D).

Although it has no important bearing on our immediate concern with vasoconstriction, this is a convenient place to call attention to some differences between the two divisions of the *autonomic nervous system*. The *sympathetic division* (which mediates peripheral vasoconstriction) has short preganglionic fibers and long postganglionic fibers, which originate in the cells of the *sympathetic chain*. For the sake of simplicity, Figure 4.1C shows only one ganglion and only a small segment of the spinal cord. Actually, there is a chain of ganglia (the sympathetic chain) on each side of the spinal cord, along its entire length. The reader must bear in mind that these diagrams in Figure 4.1C and 4.1D are greatly simplified. The *parasympathetic division*, on the other hand, has long preganglionic fibers and short postganglionic fibers. Sympathetic functions are called *adrenergic* since noradrenalin (resembling adrenalin) is the transmitter substance at the junction between the postganglionic cell and the organs (smooth and cardiac muscles), whereas parasympathetic functions (for example, slowing of the heart) are called *cholinergic* since acetylcholine is the usual

Figure 4.1B *Vasoconstriction: The way a blood vessel reduces its inside diameter (lumen).* The diagram on the left illustrates six stages (A–F) in the constriction of a small artery. For these six stages there are corresponding photographs, which were taken by means of a special technique that gives us an accurate picture of how a blood vessel (here a small artery, about one millimeter outside diameter) changes during the process of constriction. The wall of a small artery is very thin in the normal (or relatively dilated) state. (See diagram and photograph for Stage A.) In full constriction the wall of the blood vessel is much thicker. (See diagram and photograph for Stage F.) The photograph and diagram on the right show the *smooth* muscle cells (black elongated structures) inside the walls of the artery that cause constriction when they contract. This kind of muscle is called *smooth* to distinguish it from the *striate* (striped) or *skeletal* muscles, which were described in Figure 1.1A and in Chapter III. Smooth and skeletal muscles both contract (shorten), but smooth muscles contract more slowly than do skeletal muscles. When the smooth muscle cells inside the blood vessel contract, the tension produced has as its main effect the restructuring of the wall of the blood vessel, making it much thicker, causing the lumen to be reduced to about 25 percent of normal. (After Van Citters, Wagner, & Rushmer, Architecture of small arteries during vasoconstriction. *Circulation Research*, 1962, *10*, 668–675. By permission of The American Heart Association, Inc.)

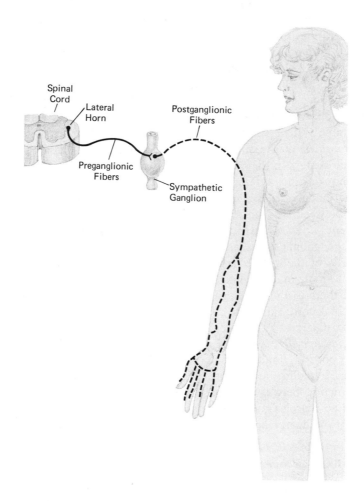

Figure 4.1C *Vasoconstrictor nerve fibers to the skin of the hand and arm.* Trace the broken line from the hand up the arm and over to the sympathetic *ganglion* (a group of nerve cell bodies located outside the brain and spinal cord, that is, outside the *central nervous system*). Broken lines represent *postganglionic* fibers (going from the ganglion to the smooth muscle cells). When activated by certain fibers coming from the ganglion, the smooth muscle cells inside the blood vessel contract, narrowing the lumen of the blood vessel in the way Figure 4.1B describes. Postganglionic neurons are activated by preganglionic neurons (motoneurons) whose cells lie in the spinal cord. (Solid line represents axons of preganglionic neurons.) The input to the preganglionic neurons (motoneurons in the spinal cord) comes from higher up in the brain (from that part of the midbrain that is part of the supraspinal motor system, as explained in Chapter III). The hypothalamus and related limbic system structures play a key role in vasoconstriction, through the pattern of neuronal impulses that they send into the midbrain.

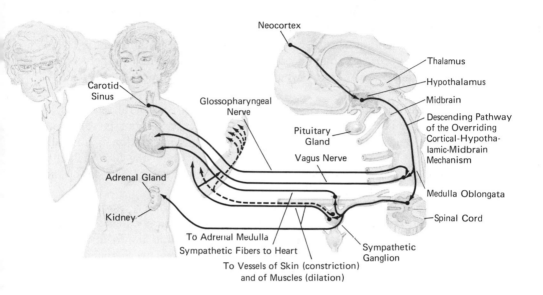

Figure 4.1D   *Neural controls of cardiovascular reactions.*   The neural pathways that were shown in Figure 4.1C are shown again here. Follow these pathways from the spinal cord to the sympathetic ganglion (via the broken lines) to the vessels of the skin in the arm and hand. This is the skin vasoconstrictor reaction to cold. In anger or in an emergency reaction, vasoconstriction in the skin is activated as part of a pattern of physiological reactions that include *dilation* of the blood vessels in the muscles (represented in the diagram by the solid lines) and increased heart rate and blood pressure. When anger subsides, or when the emergency reaction ceases, the carotid sinus mechanism operates to slow the heart and to decrease blood pressure. The reflex pathway is from carotid sinus pressoreceptors to the carotid sinus nerve, joining the glossopharyngeal nerve to the lower brain stem, and the cardiovascular centers in the medulla oblongata. From the medulla oblongata, impulses go via the vagus nerve to the heart causing it to slow down. During an emergency reaction or during a strong emotional reaction (for example, anger) the carotid sinus mechanism is overridden by a cortical-hypothalamic-midbrain mechanism so that heart rate and blood pressure remain high (see text for explanation).

transmitter substance at the final junction. For future reference it may be noted that adrenalin, which is a product of the medullary (inner) part of the adrenal glands, can be injected into the blood stream in order to speed up the heart rate and "mimic" other sympathetic activations. The effects of such injections on behavior, which have been studied by psychologists, will be dealt with later.

To return now to the question of peripheral vasoconstriction in relation to the control of body temperature, we may consider what is known concerning hypothalamic participation in this function. It seems likely that the hypothalamus participates in at least two parts of the process. First, the anterior (preoptic) hypothalamic area contains neurons that fire at a faster rate when cooled. A receptor that is situated in the brain is called a *central receptor*. Chapter VI deals in some detail with another central receptor: the osmoreceptor, which is exceedingly important in relation to thirst.

Central receptors for *cooling*, in concert with peripheral receptors in the skin, monitor temperature changes. This sensory input is somehow integrated, and although the precise nature of this integration is not well understood, it appears to be another function in which the hypothalamus (probably in its more posterior area) participates. (For location of the posterior hypothalamus, see M in Figure 3.16.)

From our discussion of pain in the preceding chapter, it will be clear that painful cooling of the extremities is far more complicated than mere transmission of intense receptor excitation. One should try to understand pain here by applying the same general principles that were stated in the preceding discussion of skeletal-muscle pains.

The posterior hypothalamus, as stated earlier, is important in relation to preparation for strong actions (such as angry attacks on another person). The sensory input for anger involves a complex perception of a social situation. It obviously lacks the relative simplicity of skin cooling, the first link in the chain of neural events that we were considering in relation to temperature regulation. To speak of a vasoconstriction that is "emotion related" is simply a convenient shorthand expression to distinguish it from vasoconstriction that is associated with something else, such as exposure to a cold environment. It does not explain anything.

Lili's cold hands were associated mainly with her emotional reactions, apparently. However, other patients suffer severe pain from cold hands, in which the pathologically strong vasoconstrictor reaction is triggered by either cold or emotion, and is especially severe when both conditions are present simultaneously. This appears to be the typical situation in Raynaud's disease, which is much more common in women than in men (Graham, 1972).

COMBINED EFFECTS OF ENVIRONMENTAL COOLING AND EMOTION

Mrs. R, a woman in her thirties, had been married and divorced twice. Her first husband, whom she married at the age of sixteen, mistreated and beat her. She divorced him after five years, resuming her work in a dress factory and performing as a professional dancer. There was one child from this marriage.

Mrs. R was twenty-two when she married the second time. After four happy years, this marriage turned out badly, too. It was during the second pregancy in this marriage that her husband began to give her less money for the household. Mrs. R became worried and hostile toward her husband. It was at this time that she first began to experience extreme discomfort from her fingers: painful attacks, which were more frequent and more severe during exposure to cold. The persistently severe symptom of pathologically strong vasoconstriction (feelings of cold and pain in the hands) is called Raynaud's disease after the French physician who described it in 1862.

Commencing with the disputes over the household budget, the marriage deteriorated. Mrs. R refused intercourse. Three months after the birth of the child her husband left her. About six months later there was reconciliation and another pregancy. But difficulties recurred and the husband left again. This time Mrs. R refused to consider reconciliation. She and the children lived in poverty because her two former husbands failed to provide sufficient support.

Mrs. R's condition was investigated in the laboratory, using procedures like those used with Lili. However, Mrs. R's condition was more severe: emotional reaction during interview produced great pain in Mrs. R's fingers. Furthermore, the combined factors of environmental cooling and emotional reaction are evident in Figure 4.2.

In other investigations of Mrs. R, it was found that when room temperature was lowered to 41° Fahrenheit, temperature alone produced pain. At a moderately cool environmental temperature (around 68° Fahrenheit), although temperature alone did not precipitate a painful attack, it was much easier for an emotional reaction to do so than in a warmer room.

Because she had so little money, Mrs. R was forced to live in a poorly heated apartment. This cold place and frequent emotional upsets combined to produce her symptoms. Mittelmann and Wolff reproduced these two conditions (cold and emotion) in the laboratory in order to demonstrate their effectiveness in making the symptoms appear.

Like the tension headaches described in the preceding chapter, blood-vessel constriction in Raynaud's disease is a specific reaction that can be activated in emotional situations. Here we have another example of close agreement between the patient's subjective complaint and objective physiological reactions observed in the laboratory.

Why do some patients suffer most from tension headaches and others from some other symptom like cold hands (or Raynaud's disease)? This is a question to which there is no simple answer. Part of the answer may lie in structural differences from person to person, which make one kind of muscle, organ, or neural mechanism particularly susceptible to over-reaction. It is well to keep in mind, incidentally, that patients often have more than one bodily symptom, although generally there is one that stands out as much more distressing than all the others.

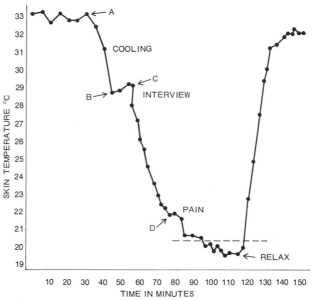

Figure 4.2 *Combined effects of environmental cooling and emotional reaction on skin temperature.* Mrs. R complains of severe pain in fingers following combined effects of environmental cooling and emotional reaction. Both conditions produce constriction of blood vessels in the hand. Procedure for measuring skin temperature with radiometer is the same as that described for Lili. Between *A* and *B* on the chart of skin temperature, part of Mrs. R's clothing is removed in a cool room. Cooling the body in this way produces a drop in skin temperature of the hand. At *B* there is transient halt to the temperature drop. At *C* Mrs. R is drawn into discussion of her illness and of her poverty, the result of ill treatment by her two former husbands. Skin temperature drops sharply again, and at *D* Mrs. R complains bitterly of pain. When the patient relaxes, skin temperature rises. (After Mittelmann & Wolff, Affective states and skin temperature: Experimental study of subjects with "cold hands" and Raynaud's syndrome. *Psychosomatic Medicine*, 1939, *1*, 271–292.)

Again, there is a specificity about the physiological reaction. For instance, Mittelmann and Wolff, who worked with Lili, Mrs. R, and other patients with cold hands, repeated their procedures with patients suffering from other bodily symptoms (for example, gastric ulcers), but not cold hands. Although interview activated strong emotions, drop in skin temperature of the hands was slight. Note that it did occur, however. Remember that vasoconstriction in the hands is part of a normal emotional reaction (involving action or preparation for action). Again, it is the degree of reaction that is important.

It should also be mentioned that when Mittelmann and Wolff interviewed their Raynaud disease patients in a comfortably warm room and on topics that were not emotion-producing, the blood vessels in their hands did not constrict. This was confirmed by the fact that the temperature readings from the radiometer remained at the same moderately high level all through the interview.

It is a common clinical assumption among physicians that Raynaud-disease sufferers often show their symptoms in emotional situations. The laboratory findings of Mittelmann and Wolff provide a solid objective basis for this assumption. Their findings have been confirmed and extended by D. T. Graham (see Graham, 1972, for a review).

D. T. Graham and co-workers have made a careful study of emotional situations that produce Raynaud-type symptoms. They concluded that the most effective situations were those that made the person want to take action (often hostile action) against another person who was behaving in an unacceptable way. It seems likely that this kind of emotional reaction would activate the mechanism described in Figure 4.1D. In short, the constriction of the blood vessels in the skin is probably an integral part of this overall mechanism that is designed for action.

Being constantly exposed to life situations that engender an attitude of hostility in an individual may well make that individual prone to Raynaud's disease. Other factors to consider are structural idiosyncrasies (as previously mentioned), and personality features (such as proneness to react with hostility).

All of these factors, and doubtless many others, enter into the development of any specific symptom, whether it be cold hands, tension headaches, high blood pressure, or some other bodily complaint. It is important to realize that symptom specificity is a multifactor problem. How much weight one attaches to each factor depends on how he interprets the many relevant research findings from investigations of a wide variety of symptoms. Buss's (1966) comprehensive summary of these findings is a significant contribution. Buss stresses the importance of laboratory research and physiological recordings.

We go on now to additional findings from our laboratory and elsewhere, which add further objective proof that patients' subjective bodily complaints have a real basis in specific physiological manifestations. We refer to evidence that patients with specific bodily complaints show clear physiological overreactions that also are specific, that is, localized to the parts of the body (or physiological mechanisms) corresponding to the symptoms.

SYMPTOM SPECIFICITY

One of the earliest experiments designed to investigate symptom specificity was done in our laboratory (Malmo & Shagass, 1949). We asked all the seventy-four patients in our psychiatric Institute at that time to participate, and there was complete cooperation. From reading each case history, we noted, first, whether or not the patient complained of discomfort in the region of the head. The complaints of this kind were chiefly of the muscle-tension variety that were described in Chapter III: for example, complaints of distressing tension (tightness) in the neck.

Second, it was noted whether or not the patients had complaints involving the heart, for example, tachycardia (fast beating of the heart), chest pains, or feelings of pressure near the heart, and palpitations (fluttering sensations around the heart).

We shall refer to these two kinds of symptoms as "head complaints" and "heart complaints." Forty-seven patients had head complaints, and twenty-seven patients did not. Thirty-four patients had heart complaints, and forty did not. There were twenty-seven patients in the group of seventy-four that had both complaints.

Heart rate, respiration, and muscle potentials from the neck were recorded continuously during our thermal pain test (described in Chapter II).

To demonstrate symptom specificity, it was necessary, first, to show that the group with head complaints were more inclined to react with increased neck muscle contraction than headache-free patients. Furthermore, in order to show that the overreaction was specific to the muscles and not merely part of a general physiological overreaction, it was necessary to show that the two groups were similar in their other physiological reactions, such as those involving the heart.

To demonstrate symptom specificity, it was also necessary to show that, compared with the headache-prone group, the group with heart complaints were more inclined to react with increased disturbances in heart rate and respiration (breathing and heart action are often closely related). Again, in order to show that the overreaction was specific to the muscles and not merely part of a general physiological overreaction, it was necessary to show that the two groups were similar in their other physiological reactions, such as those involving the skeletal muscles.

Excessive muscle-potential activity was quantified by adding the number of set time periods in which large bursts of activity appeared. Figure 4.3A shows the percentage distributions of muscle-potential scores of this group, compared with the group with no head complaints. It is evident that the group with head complaints had more frequent muscle

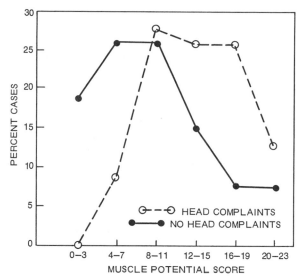

Figure 4.3A *Muscle-potential scores.* Group of patients with complaints of head-aches, and related muscle-tension discomfort in head and neck, show more bursts of muscle potentials during thermal pain test than patients without these complaints. Graphs show, for example that none of the head-complaint patients had scores as low as 3, whereas nearly 20 percent of the group without headache complaints had scores this low. (From Malmo & Shagass, Physiologic study of symptom mechanisms in psychiatric patients under stress. *Psychosomatic Medicine*, 1949, *11*, 25–29.)

potential discharges from the neck muscles than the other group of patients. The difference was statistically reliable.

Results from heart rate and heart-rate variability (corrected for age and sex factors) were also positive (see Figure 4.3B). Both heart rate and heart-rate variability were higher in the group of thirty-four patients with heart complaints than in the other group of forty patients with no heart complaints.

The measure of respiratory variability reflected deviation in rate or amplitude from each patient's prestimulation average. Close physiological relations between breathing and heart action were previously noted. Again the results were positive: the group with heart complaints showed sig-nificantly greater variations in their breathing than the group without heart complaints. As a matter of fact, only the patients with heart complaints showed extreme unsteadiness of respiration.

The evidence for physiological specificity was further strengthened by the finding that the groups positive and negative for head complaints did not differ significantly in heart rate and respiration, and that the groups positive and negative for heart complaints showed approximately equal muscle-potential scores.

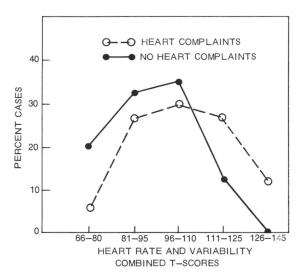

Figure 4.3B *Heart rate and variability.* Group of patients with heart complaints show higher and more variable heart rate in thermal-pain test than patients without heart complaints. *T* scores make it possible to combine scores validly. Scores for heart rate and heart-rate variability have been combined. (From Malmo & Shagass, Physiologic study of symptom mechanisms in psychiatric patients under stress. *Psychosomatic Medicine*, 1949, *11*, 25–29.)

It is important to bear in mind that all these differences were obtained even though less than 10 percent of the patients experienced their symptoms at the time of testing.

From these results (which were later essentially confirmed in our laboratory with a different group of fifty-four psychiatric patients) we concluded that the recorded disturbance appeared specific to the physiological system associated with the complaint. And, to repeat, we found that this physiological disturbance could be objectively demonstrated even though, in most instances, the subjective symptom was not experienced at the time of testing. It appeared that patients who were prone to a particular symptom characteristically reacted to the thermal pain test by bringing into play the specific physiological mechanism underlying the symptom.

As previously mentioned, symptom specificity has been confirmed by later work in our laboratory. This principle has also been confirmed by a number of other research workers, and there is general agreement that it is sound (see reviews by Buss, 1966; Engel, 1972; Goldstein, 1972; and Sternbach, 1966). Engel and co-workers, who are among the most productive researchers in this field, brought the principle of symptom specificity to bear on rheumatoid arthritis (chronic inflammation of multiple joints accompanied by pain, limitation of movement, and deformity), and hypertension (high blood pressurse).

Rheumatoid Arthritics Compared with Hypertensives

Moos and Engel (1962) investigated the muscular pains of rheumatoid arthritis, using electromyography. They placed the EMG electrodes on the muscle group that had been giving the rheumatoid arthritic the most pain during the past week. They placed the other pair of EMG electrodes on a muscle group that had always been pain-free. Another group of patients with high blood pressure had no muscle pains. Their EMG electrodes were placed so they corresponded to the placements in the group of rheumatoid arthritics, thus ensuring valid comparisons between the two groups. Blood pressure was recorded from both groups. The investigators made their recordings during a verbal test that was designed to be emotion-producing.

Findings again supported the principle of symptom specificity. Muscle potentials were higher in the arthritics' painful muscles than they were in the corresponding muscles of the hypertensives. As expected, muscle-potential levels in arthritics' pain-free muscles were similar to the hypertensives.

The investigators also looked at how adaptable the patients were in their physiological reactions. Once again, when the two groups were compared, the results during the test were in accord with the principle of symptom specificity. The hypertensives were more adaptable by the measure of muscle tension, and the arthritics were more adaptable by the measure of blood pressure. The hypertensives' muscles relaxed progressively while the arthritics' muscles remained tense throughout the session. Conversely, the hypertensives' blood pressure remained elevated when the arthritics' blood pressure was falling. In other words, the specific overreaction of the symptom mechanism in each group persisted throughout the session.

INDIVIDUAL DIFFERENCES IN PHYSIOLOGICAL REACTIONS OF NORMAL PERSONS TO EMOTIONAL SITUATIONS

Many normal persons show specificity in their physiological reactions. Schnore (1959) is one of several investigators who have drawn this conclusion from their research. As one of the conditions designed to be emotion-producing, Schnore used the tracking test with loud noise that was described in the preceding chapter; and he increased emotional intensity of the situation still more by threatening to punish with electric shock if performance was poor (although, in fact, no shocks were ever given). During the test, Schnore recorded a wide variety of physiological reactions from forty-three young men, tested one at a time.

Schnore was also interested in determining whether (a) the kind of situation and (b) the intensity of the emotion-producing conditions would affect the results of his experiments. Therefore, in addition to the tracking procedure (described earlier), he employed a difficult arithmetic task under unpleasant conditions, in which the person was frequently criticized for errors or for taking too long. He created two low-arousal conditions by lowering emotional arousal of the situations: he omitted the distracting noises and threats of shock from tracking, and he made the arithmetic test easier and less stressful. There were thus four conditions: (1) high-arousal tracking, (2) low-arousal tracking, (3) high-arousal arithmetic, and (4) low-arousal arithmetic. Muscular exertion in the four situations was similar because, in the arithmetic conditions, the person held the tracking knob so that his arm muscles were under tension, as they were in tracking.

The graphs in Figure 4.4 are typical of Schnore's findings. Forty-six of the forty-seven men had their own idiosyncratic physiological patterns which repeated themselves four times (that is, in each of the four conditions). It is quite normal, then, for a person to have his own physiological pattern of reaction in an emotion-producing situation. However, when any one reaction (for example, muscle-tension rise in neck) becomes excessive, and this reaction occurs time after time, discomfort may develop (for example, tension headache).

Generally, persons with heart complaints of the kind we were considering earlier in this chapter do not have heart disease. Careful examination by a cardiologist usually turns out negative. It therefore appears that a person can be a specific "heart reactor" without this having serious (life and death) consequences. What makes him a "heart reactor" could well be an idiosyncracy in his nervous system. Given a sound heart, then, strong or slightly irregular central activation, at times, might produce alarming sensations in a person without signifying a serious heart condition. However, an individual with a defective heart, who is also a peak "heart reactor" (like Schnore's Subject No. 4 in Figure 4.4) may be particularly vulnerable in emotion-producing situations. This would seem to be a topic well worth investigation.

The Laceys, among the first to tackle the specificity problem, appear to have been the only workers, thus far, to succeed in finding evidence that individual physiological patterns persist over time, in normal persons. They (Lacey & Lacey, 1962) tested twenty boys and seventeen girls (from seven to seventeen years of age) and then retested them four years later.

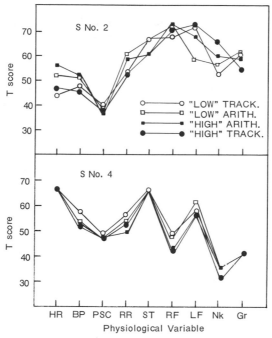

Figure 4.4 *Patterns of physiological levels for two of Schnore's subjects.* Subject number 2 is designated S2 and Subject number 4, S4. Subject 2's pattern is different from Subject 4's, but within each subject the patterns are very similar in the four different conditions: (1) high-arousal tracking, (2) low-arousal tracking, (3) high-arousal arithmetic, and (4) low-arousal arithmetic. Conversion to *T* scores makes it possible to compare different physiological functions, which are necessarily measured in different units. Physiological measures are as follows: heart rate (HR), systolic blood pressure (BP), palmar skin conductance (PSC), respiration rate (RR), skin temperature (ST), EMG from right forearm (RF), EMG from left forearm (LF), EMG from neck (Nk), and grip pressure (Gr). A *T* score near 50 means that on that measure the person was near the average for the group of 47 men on that one condition of the experiment (for example, easy arithmetic). Subject No. 2 for example (top graph) is repeatedly below average in palmar skin conductance (signifying dry palms), about average in heart rate, but consistently above average in right forearm muscle tension. The other man (Subject number 4, bottom graph) is below average in right forearm EMG but well above average in heart rate. These and other differences between the two men hold up across all four conditions.

The high-arousal conditions produced greater physiological activation (for example, higher muscle tension) than low-arousal conditions. But the graphs do not show this because of the way that the *T* scores are determined. A *T* score shows how far the individual is from the group average *in a given condition.* An average score is invariably assigned a value of 50. For example, the group averages for low- and high-arousal tracking were 38.3 and 49.9 microvolts respectively (a highly significant difference). But the *same T* score would be assigned to an individual with an overall muscle tension level of 38.3 in *low*-arousal tracking and to an individual with an overall muscle tension level of 49.9 in *high*-arousal tracking. (From Schnore, Individual patterns of physiological activity as a function of task differences and degree of arousal. *Journal of Experimental Psychology,* 1959, *58,* 117–128. Copyright 1959 by the American Psychological Association and reproduced by permission.)

They had the children take the "cold pressor test" (immersing the foot in ice water for 80 seconds), which is painful, and normally causes blood pressure to rise. They recorded systolic and diastolic blood pressures, heart rate, heart-rate variability, and palmar conductance (chiefly an index of palmar sweating). Similarities in individual physiological patterns were great enough from test to retest to be significant.[3]

To return for a moment to the discussion of psychiatric patients who complain of "heart symptoms," the evidence strongly suggests that as long as these patients have their symptoms, their hearts are overreactive in emotion-producing situations. It would be interesting to follow these patients over a period of time in order to determine whether their physiological reactions would become more normal when they were free of complaints.

We have already noted a parallel observation for tension headache in Chapter III. The forehead muscle EMGs of the woman with forehead-tension headaches were at a much lower level, later in treatment, when her headaches were diminishing.

PROSPECTS FOR VOLUNTARY CONTROL OF AUTONOMIC FUNCTIONS

Our patient with the painful tension in her forehead muscles improved with psychiatric treatment, and part of this improvement was reflected in much lower EMGs from the forehead muscles.

We did not try to reduce forehead tension directly. Relaxation in forehead muscle tension was part of general improvement following comprehensive treatment. This is as it should be, of course. The psychiatrist treats the patient, and not merely a symptom. Recently, there have been some developments that raise our hopes that learning (or "feedback") techniques may be useful adjuncts to treatment of patients with tension headaches and other bodily complaints. The reader is warned at the outset, however, to exercise critical control over premature enthusiasm for these developments. Fascinating as they are, much further research is required before we can be really sure of our ground.

Feedback (or "Biofeedback")

Feedback training as applied to tension headache may be visualized as follows. Imagine our patient with the tense forehead muscles seated in front of a meter, like the one in our tracking test (see Chapter III). For

---

[3] The reader who is interested in further details about specificity of physiological reactions should consult Sternbach's (1966) book.

feedback training, only one meter is required. The needle on this meter registers tension in the patient's forehead muscles.[4]

By watching the needle, the patient has moment-to-moment information about her forehead tension. Now her doctor asks her to try to bring the needle down the scale by relaxing her forehead muscles. Trying various ways of relaxing the forehead muscles, and finding a way to move the needle down the scale, would be learning by feedback.

The suggestion (Malmo, 1970) that EMG feedback might be useful in treating persons with tension headaches has recently received support. There is strong evidence now that this technique actually works. Quite independently, at the University of Colorado Medical Center, a pilot study was carried out to test feedback technique in treating patients with headaches due to sustained contraction of head or neck muscles (Budzynski, Stoyva, & Adler, 1970). Positive results from the pilot study were followed up with a systematic study by Budzynski, Stoyva, Adler, and Mullaney (1973). In these studies, the feedback was auditory. In the main study, the information concerning EMG (tension) levels in the frontalis muscles was provided by click rate. Through headphones the person heard a train of discrete clicks. When EMG activity was high, the click rate was fast. When EMG activity decreased, the click rate also decreased. The person attempted to relax as thoroughly as possible, aided by the information feedback provided by the clicks.

In the main study there were eighteen persons, all with complaints of frequent tension headaches over a long period. These persons were divided into three groups of six persons each. Group A persons received accurate information about their frontalis tension from the click rate fed back to them through the earphones. Group B (a "pseudofeedback" group) heard clicks, but the click rate did *not* provide accurate information about the changes in frontalis muscle tension. They listened to feedback signals that had been tape-recorded from Group A. Persons in both groups were instructed to practice relaxation of their frontalis muscles twice a day at home or at work (in the absence of any feedback equipment). Persons in Groups A and B attended two feedback sessions per week over a nine-week period. Persons in Group C received no treatment at all.

The results showed that frontalis EMG levels in Group A (accurate feedback group) fell to less than 40 percent of initial baseline values. In Group B (inaccurate or "pseudofeedback" group), on the other hand, EMG levels stayed up at about 80 percent of the baseline values. At the

---

[4] It was convenient to illustrate the principle of EMG feedback by means of this visual monitoring model. Actually, auditory monitoring is generally used for this purpose.

end of the three-month follow-up period the difference between the groups was even greater, and was highly reliable statistically.

Reports of headache in Group A were significantly lower than in Groups B and C toward the end of the nine-week training period. Persons in Group A, but not those in Group B, characteristically showed a sharply reduced use of medication. In short, persons in the accurate feedback group showed diminished headache activity, greatly decreased drug usage, and significantly reduced frontalis EMG levels relative to those of the two control groups.

Stoyva and Budzynski (in press) reported the results of subsequent work. Since the controlled outcome study was completed, over sixty persons have undergone the training. Seventy-five percent of these persons have shown substantial reductions in headache activity, whereas fewer than 25 percent of the twelve controls have shown substantial improvement.

In the same report Stoyva and Budzynski also made some interesting qualitative observations. Persons in training "typically passed through several stages in terms of their ability to use a 'cultivated' relaxation response to reduce headache activity. At first they were able to relax only with deliberate effort. Later, the relaxation response became easier to do, even when the patient felt under some pressure." Finally, with some persons, "the relaxation response appeared to have become virtually an automatic reaction, no longer requiring conscious effort."

Lang (1970) used feedback in teaching college students to control their heart rates. The student watched a small lighted disc on a screen. When the student's heart rate coincided with his average heart rate (for example, 60 beats per minute, or one second between beats), the spot of light appeared on a vertical line in the middle of the screen. When his heart beat at a faster rate (less than one second between beats), the spot of light moved to the left; when at a slower rate (more than one second between beats), the light moved to the right.

The students were told to keep the spot within a narrow "road." The apparatus was like a driving-skill booth at an amusement park: the students learned by feedback to "drive" their own hearts. The learning worked well. The students soon were skilled at keeping the light "on the road," and they improved still more with practice.

What the students were really learning to do, of course, was to make their heart rhythms more regular. The relatively slight irregularities of the heartbeat in healthy students are well within safe limits. But heart patients with dangerous arrhythmias have apparently improved with feedback treatment. Engel and co-workers have used a technique similar in principle to Lang's, in working with patients suffering from serious irregularities of the heartbeat (see Collier, 1971).

Engel's apparatus has red, yellow, and green lights arranged like traffic lights. These lights are connected with an apparatus like Lang's, which continuously monitors heart rate and makes the lights change according to the changes in heart rate. (Engel uses an electrocardiograph and a specially programmed computer.) Red means the heart rate is too fast and green that it is too slow. Keeping the yellow light on, like staying on the "road" in Lang's apparatus, is the goal for the heart patient. The results thus far have been encouraging; like the headache patients, some of these heart patients appear to retain their learning, so that they can control the regularity of their heartbeats away from the machine. Many more observations are needed, however, before we can be confident that feedback technique will have useful applications for a significant number of individuals.

How do people learn to bring heart rate and other autonomic functions under control? Apparently they themselves do not know, or at least they cannot put it into words. Conscious changes in breathing can affect heart rate; but Lang and associates were careful to do the necessary control experiments to make sure their subjects were not controlling their heart rates through changes in their breathing patterns. Only by much further research will we be able to interpret these phenomena and judge the generality of their occurrence.

Work on feedback training received a tremendous boost from reports of remarkable findings by Miller, DiCara, and their associates, who conducted a series of experiments with rats. An account of some of their positive results follows. However, a recent development should be borne in mind. Miller (in press) has reported that subsequent attempts to replicate some of these experiments have failed to produce such reliable results. With this in mind, and in the realization that early reports of successes with a new clinical treatment have in the past often been premature, Miller urges the greatest caution against drawing premature conclusions. Despite some negative results, there are still many reports that encourage further extensive research in this general area.

In early experiments in their series, Miller, DiCara, and their associates found that rats paralyzed by curare learned to speed or to slow their heart rates (from their normal rates), depending on which kind of change was rewarded. They used brain stimulation as reward.[5] They reported making the rat's heart rate rise to levels above its normal pretraining rate by rewarding it with brain stimulation each time the heart rate increased spontaneously. They also reported that they could produce

---

[5] Olds and Milner were the first to find that electrical stimulation in certain areas of the brain has a rewarding effect. (For a recent review, see Milner, 1970.)

the opposite effect, slowing, by rewarding the rat each time its heart rate slowed.[6] They used EMG recording to monitor paralysis by curare.

From the results of further experiments, Miller, DiCara, and co-workers reported that the same kind of training produced changes in other autonomic functions. These included stomach contractions, urine formation, blood pressure, and changes in the lumens of blood vessels (*vaso-motor* changes). In one particularly remarkable experiment, DiCara and Miller reported success in having rats blush one ear (*vasodilate*) and blanch (*vasoconstrict*) the other. (For a review of this series of experiments, see Miller, 1969.)

USEFULNESS OF AUTONOMIC FUNCTIONS

While it would be an advantage in many cases to gain voluntary control over a troublesome condition such as hypertension, it is, of course, a distinct advantage to have autonomic mechanisms go on working without requiring our attention.

One of the most important regulatory mechanisms is the one that prevents the condition of chronically high blood pressure, known as *hypertension*. Extreme hypertension can produce fatal heart failure.

An autonomic reflex normally prevents blood pressure from remaining at high levels over long periods of time. The main receptors for this reflex are in the *carotid sinus*, an enlarged section of the carotid artery, going to the head. (See Figure 4.1D.) These receptors (called *presso-receptors* or *baroreceptors*) are pressure-sensitive. They change their rate of firing with changes in the arterial blood pressure: the higher the pressure, the greater their rate of firing. The pressoreceptors discharge their impulses into the carotid sinus nerve, joining the glossopharyngeal nerve, which enters the brain stem, and goes to cardiovascular centers in the *medulla oblongata* (a part of the base of the brain with connections to *autonomic ganglia*, as explained earlier in this chapter). From the medulla, impulses go via the vagus nerve to the heart, causing it to slow down. The vagus nerve is part of the *parasympathetic* nervous system. The *sympathetic* nervous system has opposite effects. When dominant, it causes speeding of the heart. Strong discharge of impulses from the presso-receptors makes the parasympathetic division dominant. Consequently,

---

[6] These experiments are complicated somewhat by the fact that brain stimulation that is rewarding produces heart-rate changes directly, apparently by stimulating autonomic mechanisms for heart-rate slowing. Since the experiments in Miller's laboratory produced learned heart-rate changes in both directions, speeding as well as slowing, this complication seems to be controlled for. Moreover, Miller and co-workers used incentives other than brain stimulation successfully. However, because it is interesting, we should keep in mind the fact that brain stimulations in these areas produce various autonomic changes directly.

sympathetic firing to the heart and blood vessels decreases. Lumens of the blood vessels in the skin widen (*vasodilate*). These and other physiological changes, which were initially set into action by the pressoreceptors responding to increased arterial blood pressure, work to bring blood pressure down to a normal level (for further details, see Scher, 1965).

"Emotional" Situations Override Reflex Regulation of Blood Pressure

In strong "emotion," the body's physiological mechanisms are mobilized for action. When a person faces danger, for example, heart rate and blood pressure are increased as part of the preparation for muscular exertion. Perception of danger (for example, seeing and smelling smoke) triggers these preparatory mechanisms. Blood pressure rises and remains high during the emergency. The "emergency reaction," activating cortical-hypothalamic-midbrain mechanisms (see Figure 4.1D), overrides the regulatory mechanism in the medulla.

After a brief emergency (for example, fire in wastepaper basket), with perception of danger removed, the cortical-hypothalamic-midbrain control over the medullary mechanism is likewise removed, thereby permitting this regulatory mechanism to bring blood pressure down.

Nature seems to have designed the cortical-hypothalamic-midbrain mechanism for emergencies of relatively short duration. Among the mammals it is man who has managed to produce long stressful periods for himself. As we observed in Chapter II, when people have to live under intensely stressful conditions over prolonged periods, regulatory mechanisms appear to have their set-points raised and held at the higher level much longer than is appropriate.

More than a quarter of the soldiers who had seen protracted combat in the African desert in World War II continued to have high blood pressure (as high as hypertensive patients) for several months after removal from combat (see Graham, 1972). This suggests that the set-point for the pressoreceptive-medullary control of blood pressure was raised during the protracted period of combat, under adverse climatic conditions, and then remained inappropriately high. A possible neurophysiological mechanism that could account for inappropriate "stickiness" of the set-point in regulatory mechanisms will be considered in Chapter VII.

Possibilities exist for feedback training to help some patients with chronically high blood pressure. It is evident that stressful life situations can make the cortical-hypothalamic-midbrain mechanism dominant over the regulatory pressoreceptor-medullary mechanism. Therefore, it seems reasonable that for these persons feedback training might be used to help remove this abnormal dominance, thus restoring normal regulation sooner in the poststress period than would be the case without the training. There are, for instance, encouraging positive findings of blood-pressure control with feedback in normal persons (Shapiro, Tursky, Gershon, & Stern, 1969). But, again, it is too early to be sure how successful these feedback techniques will be in helping a significant number of hypertensive patients.

SUMMARY

The *autonomic* nervous system gets its name from the fact that many of its functions operate without our having to attend to them. For example, blood vessels in our limbs constrict when we go out in a cold environment, thus assisting in the regulation of body temperature to a set-point, which is essential for health. We are usually unconscious of this vasoconstriction and its consequences. However, in Raynaud's disease the consequences of vasoconstriction are perceived as painful, and this pain is aggravated by emotional disturbances, which further increase the vasoconstriction.

Neural mechanisms mediating perception of cold were described, and special attention was called to the recent discovery of brain cells that fire at a faster rate in a cold environment. These cells were considered in relation to the concept of internal *push*, which will be considered again in Chapter V and in Chapter VI when we discuss the functions of osmoreceptors (brain cells that fire at a faster rate in cellular dehydration thirst).

Autonomic reactions such as fast beating of the heart, high blood pressure, and rapid breathing are involved in preparing for action, and they are therefore closely associated with skeletal-motor activity. Some persons are most prone to overreaction in certain autonomic functions, and these persons develop specific autonomic symptoms instead of symptoms involving the skeletal muscles (for example, tension headaches). This is an example of *symptom specificity*. Physiological response specificity is characteristic of persons generally, and each individual has his own physiological profile. This principle is well established from extensive research with normal persons.

Recently there have been some exciting developments to raise our hopes that learning (or "feedback") techniques may be useful adjuncts to treatment of patients with tension headaches and other bodily complaints including disorders of the autonomic nervous system such as high blood pressure. This active area of clinical research is one that should continue to yield important data for some time to come. At this stage of the research, it is wise to be extremely cautious about drawing premature conclusions.

Actually, it is an advantage to have autonomic regulatory mechanisms that operate without our having to think about them. For instance, the carotid sinus reflex is valuable in lowering blood pressure when it exceeds the normal level. The carotid sinus mechanism is overridden by a cortical-hypothalamic-midbrain mechanism when the individual faces an emergency requiring an energetic response. After a brief emergency, the carotid sinus mechanism regains dominance and restores normal blood pressure. However, a long stressful period with the cortical-hypothalamic-midbrain mechanism continually overriding the carotid sinus reflex, will keep blood pressure at a high level, in some instances months after the individual has been removed from the stressful environment. This "stickiness" is a special case of a general phenomenon, which was described in Chapter II with regard to chronic anxiety. In general terms, the phenomenon may be viewed as a physiological mechanism operating at an abnormally high set-point long after the environmental demands have returned to normal. This unnecessarily prolonged elevation of the set-point signifies the retention of an archaic brain mechanism, While this mechanism works well in preparing the individual for short-term emergencies, it is archaic in its "stickiness." The set-point does not come down when it should. The possible neural basis of this "stickiness" will be discussed in Chapter VII, with particular reference to chronic anxiety.

In Chapter V our interest will shift to a consideration of relatively short-term situations. The main topic will be the relations between arousal level and level of performance.

REFERENCES

Budzynski, T. H., Stoyva, J. M., & Adler, C. S. Feedback-induced muscle relaxation: Application to tension headache. *Journal of Behavior Therapy and Experimental Psychiatry*, 1970, *1*, 205–211.

Budzynski, T. H., Stoyva, J. M., Adler, C. S., & Mullaney, D. J. EMG biofeedback and tension headache: A controlled outcome study. *Psychosomatic Medicine*, 1973, *35*, 484–496.

Buss, A. H. *Psychopathology*. New York: Wiley, 1966.

Collier, B. L. Brain power. The case for bio-feedback training. *Saturday Review*, April 10, 1971. Pp. 10–58.

Engel, B. T. Response specificity. In N. S. Greenfield & R. A. Sternbach (Eds.), *Handbook of psychophysiology*. New York: Holt, Rinehart and Winston, 1972. Pp. 571–576.

Engel, B. T., & Bickford, A. F. Response specificity. Stimulus-response and individual-response specificity in essential hypertensives. *Archives of General Psychiatry*, 1961, *5*, 478–489.

Goldstein, I. B. Electromyography: A measure of skeletal muscle response. In N. S. Greenfield & R. A. Sternbach (Eds.), *Handbook of psychophysiology*. New York: Holt, Rinehart and Winston, 1972. Pp. 329–365.

Graham, D. T. Psychosomatic medicine. In N. S. Greenfield & R. A. Sternbach (Eds.), *Handbook of psychophysiology.* New York: Holt, Rinehart and Winston, 1972. Pp. 839–924.

Lacey, J. I., & Lacey, B. C. The law of initial value in the longitudinal study of autonomic constitution: Reproducibility of autonomic responses and response patterns over a four-year interval. *Annals of the New York Academy of Sciences,* 1962, *98,* 1257–1290.

Lang, P. J. Autonomic control or learning to play the internal organs. *Psychology Today,* 1970, *4,* 37–86.

Malmo, R. B. Emotions and muscle tension: The story of Anne. *Psychology Today,* 1970, *3,* 64–83.

Malmo, R. B., & Shagass, C. Physiologic study of symptom mechanisms in psychiatric patients under stress. *Psychosomatic Medicine,* 1949, *11,* 25–29.

Miller, N. E. Learning of visceral and glandular responses. *Science,* 1969, *163,* 434–445.

Miller, N. E. Applications of learning and biofeedback to psychiatry and medicine. In A. M. Freedman, H. I. Kaplan, & B. J. Sadock (Eds.), *Comprehensive textbook of psychiatry.* (2nd ed.) Baltimore: Williams & Wilkins, in press.

Milner, P. M. *Physiological psychology.* New York: Holt, Rinehart and Winston, 1970.

Mittelmann, B., & Wolff, H. G. Affective states and skin temperature: Experimental study of subjects with "cold hands" and Raynaud's syndrome. *Psychosomatic Medicine,* 1939, *1,* 271–292.

Moos, R. H., & Engel, B. T. Psychophysiological reactions in hypertensive and arthritic patients. *Journal of Psychosomatic Research,* 1962, *6,* 227–241.

Rushmer, R. F. The arterial system: Arteries and arterioles. In T. C. Ruch & H. D. Patton (Eds.), *Physiology and biophysics.* Philadelphia: W. B. Saunders, 1965. Pp. 600–616.

Scher, A. M. Control of arterial blood pressure: Measurement of pressure and flow. In T. C. Ruch & H. D. Patton (Eds.), *Physiology and biophysics.* Philadelphia: W. B. Saunders, 1965. Pp. 660–683.

Schnore, M. M. Individual patterns of physiological activity as a function of task differences and degree of arousal. *Journal of Experimental Psychology,* 1959, *58,* 117–128.

Shapiro, D., Tursky, B., Gershon, E., & Stern, M. Effects of feedback and reinforcement on the control of human systolic blood pressure. *Science,* 1969, *163,* 588–590.

Sternbach, R. A. *Principles of psychophysiology.* New York: Academic Press, 1966.

Stoyva, J. M., & Budzynski, T. H. Cultivated low arousal—an anti-stress response? In L. V. DiCara (Ed.), *Recent advances in limbic and autonomic nervous system research.* New York: Plenum (in press).

Uvnäs, B. Central cardiovascular control. In J. Field, H. W. Magoun, & V. E. Hall (Eds.), *Handbook of physiology—Neurophysiology*. Vol. II. Washington: American Physiological Society, 1960. Pp. 1131–1162.

Van Citters, R. L., Wagner, B. M., & Rushmer, R. F. Architecture of small arteries during vasoconstriction. *Circulation Research*, 1962, *10*, 668–675.

V

"Arousal"
and Performance

UNDER INTENSE EMOTION a person is liable to behave in ways that are unusual for him. Allowances are often made for what people do (or fail to do) under conditions of extreme emotional stress. Unfortunately, however, the loss of efficiency resulting from emotional overstimulation may be calamitous.

Canadian psychiatrist J. S. Tyhurst conducted field surveys in four disasters: two large apartment-house fires, a flash flood, and a fire on a crowded vacation steamship in dock. The impact of any disaster situation is typically sudden, generally causing severe fright, and making most people behave stupidly just at a time when they most need to keep their wits about them.

Tyhurst (1951) who conducted interviews with disaster survivors immediately afterwards, distinguished three main "types" within each group of survivors. The first type (12–25 percent) could be described as "cool and collected" during the acute situation. They were able to perceive things clearly and to take appropriate action. The second type (about ¾ of the survivors) were stunned and bewildered, lacked clear perception, and acted in an "automatic fashion." The third type (10–25 percent) failed to react (for example, couldn't move out of bed), as though paralyzed by fright, or else acted inappropriately, by crying, screaming, or doing foolhardy things. (One man continued to search for a missing cuff link instead of moving to save his life.)

Leaving a sinking ship in lifeboats is another situation where incredibly ineffective behavior has been observed. When the *Titanic* sank after hitting an iceberg, little more than half the number of people were saved that might have been. Some 500 persons failed to use lifeboats that were available, although a calm sea and other conditions were favorable for them to get into lifeboats during the two hours the ship was sinking.

On the torpedoed *Lusitania* many people huddled, as though paralyzed, along the rails until the ship sank. Nearly 1200 people drowned. One eighteen-year-old boy (from the "cool and collected" group) emerged as leader and did as much as one person could do to fill and launch lifeboats, proving, incidentally, that many more lives could have been saved (see Caldwell, Ranson, & Sacks, 1951).

Observers of soldiers in battle have described similarly maladaptive behavior. For instance, there is the commonly observed "panic run" in which during a shelling, the soldier deserts cover and dashes about aimlessly, exposing himself to flying shell fragments.

Military analyst Colonel S. L. A. Marshall (1947) observed that in World War II, soldiers' immobility and failure to fire in battle were common fear reactions: "When the infantryman's mind is gripped by fear, his body is captured by inertia, which is fear's Siamese twin." Marshall presents convincing evidence that failure to fire is caused by paralyzing fear (and is not merely due to the soldier's wishing to avoid exposing his position to the enemy). The following account is an example of the documentation:

> In this situation the commander, Lieutenant Colonel Robert G. Cole (later killed in action in Holland) was able to keep moving up and down along the column despite a harassing fire, and observe the attitude of all riflemen and weapons men. This was his testimony, given in the presence of the assembled battalion: "I found no way to make them continue fire. Not one man in twenty-five voluntarily used his weapon. There was no cover; they could not dig in. Therefore their only protection was to continue a fire which would make the enemy keep his head down. They had been taught this principle in training. They all knew it very well. But they could not force themselves to act upon it. When I ordered the men who were right around me to fire, they did so. But the moment I passed on, they quit. I walked up and down the line yelling, 'God damn it! Start shooting!' But it did little good. They fired only while I watched them or while some other officer stood over them (Marshall, 1947, p. 72).

These observations have some important features in common despite the fact that there are striking differences between the emergency of leaving a sinking ship and that of protecting oneself on the battlefield. In each situation the individual is exposed to a terrifying situation and, at the same time, is called on to perform efficiently.

When we consider the individuals who showed immobility in these situations, one of the first things that occurs to us, of course, is the primordial biological value of immobility ("freezing") in hiding from a predator. Here we seem to have another example of activating the vestige of an archaic brain mechanism, which is now inappropriate under "civilized" conditions; and the same may be said of the "panic run" on the battlefield.

Results of these field studies raise interesting questions, which one would like to pursue under controlled conditions of laboratory experimentation. The reader hardly needs to be reminded of the very great difficulties inherent in such pursuits. One condition of a careful experiment by Stennett (1957) was designed to reveal the impairing effect of a situation in which the individuals were threatened with strong electric shock and loss of large money bonuses if they failed to do well in a task of skill. Physiological recordings were taken in this experiment.

Stennett used an auditory tracking task similar to the one described in Chapter III. The person rotated a knob slowly back and forth with his right hand, being guided by tones heard in earphones. When he turned the knob at precisely the correct velocity, the person heard no tone in his earphones. When he turned the knob too quickly or too slowly he heard tones that informed him whether he was going too fast or too slowly and by how much. At the end of each two-minute tracking trial, the experimenter read the time-off-target from a precision electric clock.

Muscle potentials were recorded from two muscle groups of the right and left forearm. Tracking was done with the right hand under three different conditions. In the first (high-incentive) condition, Stennett offered large money bonuses for good performance and threatened the person with strong electric shock if performance dropped too low. In his second (moderate-incentive) condition, Stennett used money rewards again, but not so large as to be overstimulating; and there was no threat of shock. In the third (low-incentive) condition, the person was told that his score was not important because the real purpose of these tracking trials was calibration of the apparatus.

Figure 5.1 shows that Stennett was successful in producing muscle-tension changes that differentiated well between the three conditions. The conditions with threat of strong electric shock produced the highest muscle tension, but performance on tracking was impaired relative to that on the condition with moderate incentive, which yielded the best performance of all.

Stennett's experiment is a clear laboratory demonstration of efficiency loss associated with expectation of strong electric shock and other con-

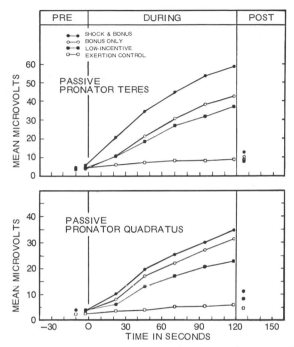

Figure 5.1 *Muscle tension from left-arm muscle groups during tracking perform-ance under three different conditions.* Note that muscle tension rises during the two-minute trial. These rises are electromyographic (EMG) gradients, which were discussed in Chapter III. The two muscle groups are pronator quadratus (wrist) and pronator teres (upper forearm). Curves are based on averages from 31 male univer-sity students. Top curve, first condition: threat of strong shock for doing poorly, and large money bonuses for doing well. Second highest curve, second condition: mod-erate incentive (encouragement with modest money bonuses and no threat of shock). Third highest curve, third condition: low-incentive (subjects were told performance scores were not important). Bottom curve: (merely holding the knob over against resistance *without* tracking) shows that in order to produce EMG gradients, the subject must perform the tracking task. EMG gradients are not produced merely by muscular exertion. Performance on tracking was best with moderate incentive. (After Stennett, The relationship of performance level to level of arousal. *Journal of Experi-mental Psychology*, 1957, *54*, 54–61. Copyright 1957 by the American Psychological Association, and reproduced by permission.)

tingencies. As mentioned earlier, this kind of laboratory demonstration is difficult to achieve. Comparing field conditions (for example, battlefield or civilian disaster) with laboratory conditions, it is first of all obvious that the latter cannot match the former in intensity of impact. Secondly, observations from field studies show the importance of individual differ-ences in degree and kind of reactions to threatening situations. Therefore the results of a laboratory experiment based on group averages must be interpreted with great caution.

The kind of difference that Stennett observed between his second and third conditions is much easier to demonstrate in the laboratory. This is the difference between a condition of moderately high incentive (optimal for performance) and a condition of low incentive (significantly below optimal for performance). In the description of Stennett's experiment, thus far only muscle-potential data from the left arm muscles have been mentioned. Other physiological data reflecting similar differences between conditions were heart rate, palmar sweating, and muscle potentials from the right arm.

We extended Stennett's battery of physiological measures, and found in a group of fifty-nine men that all the averaged measures showed significantly greater physiological activation (along with better tracking performance on the average) in going from a condition of low to one of moderate incentive (Malmo, 1965). Our measures were muscle potentials from muscles of left and right forearms, heart rate, breathing rate, and sweating on the palm and fingers of the left hand.

The muscular exertion required for low-incentive tracking is exactly the same as for high-incentive tracking. Why then should heart and breathing rate, muscle tension, and hand sweating be greater for high-than for low-incentive tracking? One possible answer is that somehow the person's autonomic nervous mechanisms react to the high-incentive situation *as though* greater muscular exertion is going to be required. In other words, the person's perception of the high-incentive situation activates neurophysiological mechanisms that prepare him for greater *muscular* exertion than is actually required (for example, to turn the knob in tracking). There is a preparation for action, something apparently related to role rehearsal.

Referring back to Chapter III, we may view this "overactivation" of the muscles and of accompanying reactions as a further sign that our brain is archaic in its overly strong facilitation on the motor system. The reader may object that for optimal tracking, a higher level of muscle tension is needed for "toning up" the muscles than the level reached in the low-motivation condition. But this objection breaks down because it cannot validly be raised against the still greater rise in muscle tension in Stennett's shock-expectation condition in which tracking was *impaired.*

Suppose we pause briefly in order to view these experimental results and the field-study observations in relation to the neuropsychology of efficiency.

Brain functioning, the basis for the organism's coping with its environment, has been shaped by external conditions existing in nature. Therefore we can expect the animal to experience difficulties when the experimenter contrives a set of experimental conditions that fail to correspond to those that "shaped" its brain. The reader who has followed the argument about the archaic nature of our brain knows that this is precisely the state of affairs in which we human beings often find ourselves. But what about animals?

An ingenious animal experiment by Broadhurst (1957) is relevant to the question raised in the preceding paragraph. Broadhurst trained rats to swim under water in a Y-shaped maze toward two lights placed behind translucent doors. By choosing the arm of the Y with the brighter light and by pushing against the door on that side, the rat could escape to the air. However, if the rat chose the wrong arm of the Y, escape was blocked by a locked door, and the rat was forced to go around to the side where the brighter light was placed. Lights were shifted from side to side randomly, so that the rat had to attend to the brightness of the lights, being unable to choose correctly merely on the basis of position (that is, going to the same side each time).

There were three levels of difficulty: (a) the easiest task, where one light was 300 times brighter than the other; (b) a task intermediate in difficulty where the ratio was 60:1, and (c) the most difficult task, where the ratio was only 15:1. There were four levels of incentive. Broadhurst varied incentive by keeping rats submerged under water for different periods of time before releasing them to swim through the maze. The four different delay periods were 0, 2, 4, and 8 seconds.

Results are shown in Figure 5.2. Being retained under water for 8 seconds without air greatly impaired the rat's learning of a difficult brightness discrimination. The neural capabilities of the rat were insufficient to manage this combination of conditions, although they were sufficient to allow moderately good learning of the difficult discrimination when the rat was kept without air in the preperiod for only 2 seconds, instead of 8. The rat's good learning performance on the *moderately* difficult discrimination even with an 8-second preperiod under water shows that this amount of time without air does not by itself prevent the rat from performing in the maze. But the *combination* of the long preperiod (which must be "frightening" to the rat) and the difficult discrimination immediately thereafter appears to be responsible for the breakdown in performance.

Finally it will be noted that *some* enforced delay under water prior to swimming had a more beneficial effect on learning than no delay at all. Looking at the whole picture then, the results are like Stennett's with the most beneficial effects on performance coming from moderate incentive.

There is an extensive literature on how performance is affected by environmental and other factors. We shall return to some of these studies later in this chapter. At this point, it will be useful to review some neuropsychological experiments involving the reticular system which, perhaps more than any other part of the brain, appears to play a key role in the mediation of these phenomena.

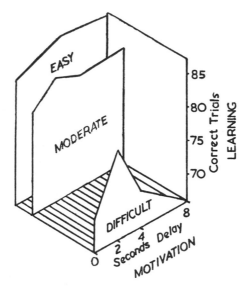

Figure 5.2 *Learning performances of rats escaping from underwater Y maze.* In order to escape, rats learn to go into the arm of the *Y* that has the brighter of the two lights. The rats are retained under water for varying periods prior to swimming in the maze. Learning was most impaired with a combination of long foreperiod under water (8 seconds) and having to make a difficult discrimination at the end of the maze. Difficulty was increased by making the two lights more alike in brightness (that is, decreasing the brightness ratio). (From Broadhurst, Emotionality and the Yerkes-Dodson law. *Journal of Experimental Psychology*, 1957, *54*, 345–352. Copyright 1957 by the American Psychological Association, and reproduced by permission.)

RETICULAR CORE OF THE BRAIN STEM

Look at the cross-hatched structure diagrammed in Figure 5.3. As recently as twenty-five years ago, the importance of the *reticular formation* was not recognized. Its tangled network (*reticular* means "netlike") was regarded by most neuroscientists as so much neural filler (like excelsior packing) mixed in with the truly important structures, which were orderly (that is, columnar) in appearance. Now, following some epoch-making discoveries commencing about twenty-five years ago and after an enormous amount of research since then, the reticular core of the brain stem is considered to be one of the most important areas of the brain.

The reticulo-spinal tracts (the descending parts of the reticular system) are an extremely important part of the motor system, which was discussed in Chapter III. These tracts originate at the level of the pons (see the figure) and go directly to the motoneurons in the ventral horn of the spinal cord (refer back to Chapter III). It will be recalled that the hypothalamus and other parts of the limbic system have no direct pro-

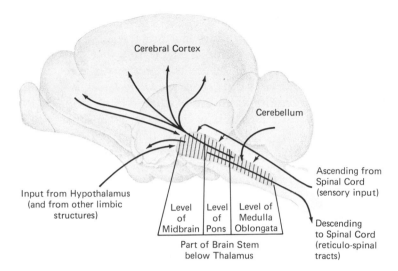

Figure 5.3 *Diagram (side or saggital view) showing some of the relations between a part of the brain stem reticular core and other parts of the brain.* The cross-hatched area represents the reticular core lying below the thalamus. This region, plus a small part of the posterior thalamic reticular formation, contains the areas from which low-threshold arousal responses can be elicited by electrical stimulation. (After Starzl, Taylor, & Magoun, Collateral afferent excitation of reticular formation of brain stem. *Journal of Neurophysiology,* 1951, *14,* 479–496.)

jections to the spinal cord. As Figure 5.3 indicates, their *efferent* outflow goes to the midbrain region and stops there. This means that the input to the midbrain reticular core from the limbic system enters into neuronal transactions that involve inputs from many other parts of the brain (including the neocortex) and from sensory pathways ascending in the spinal cord.

Projections from the reticular core go to many parts of the brain, including the hypothalamus and the cerebral cortex. The projections to the cerebral cortex from the reticular core were involved in an epoch-making discovery by Moruzzi and Magoun (1949), which brought the reticular core into the spotlight. The Moruzzi and Magoun discovery may be illustrated by reference to Figure 3.9. Look first at the lower EEG tracings (E–H) of alpha activity, which is associated with a state of quiet relaxation. Moruzzi and Magoun discovered that animals showing this synchronized EEG pattern could be made to show the desynchronized fast-frequency beta pattern (A–D in the figure) by electrically stimulating their reticular core. At the same time, the animal showed signs of *behavioral arousal.* The EEG change that they observed is called EEG *activation,* which had been known for some time. Persons show a change in their EEGs from synchronized alpha to desynchronized beta when they are asked to pay attention to something, or are alerted in some way. The importance of the Moruzzi and Magoun discovery (now replicated countless times) lay in their demonstration of the role that the reticular core plays in this behavioral change. Since their discovery, the reticular system is frequently referred to as the *reticular activating system.*

Here we may consider again the possible role of feedback from the muscles, which was discussed in Chapter III in connection with Hodes' experiment with curare. It will be recalled that Hodes believed that the cerebellum was involved in relaying impulses generated by muscle receptors. Figure 5.3 shows an input from the cerebellum to the reticular core, which likely would be a most effective means of relaying neural activation on to the neocortex. Curare, in eliminating muscle contraction and feedback from muscle receptors, would eliminate this source of activation, which would be one way of accounting for Hodes' finding that, with curare, his animals' EEGs changed from a desynchronized to a synchronized pattern.

Since we have turned our attention back to Chapter III, this will be a convenient time to consider EMG gradients in relation to the reticular system. Recall that the activated (beta) EEG pattern in subjects prior to their hearing a story predicted those subjects who, during listening to the story, would show good EMG gradients. Although admittedly speculative, this suggests some possible connection between the subject's EEG pattern, his EMG gradient, and his *involvement* with the story. (Refer again to the text of Chapter III explaining correlations between these three items.)

In short, from the foregoing and from some other observations, which were covered in Chapter III, it seems reasonable now to suggest (in a very tentative way) how the reticular core might be involved in EMG gradients.

First of all, it should be stated that an activated EEG pattern from the neocortex merely indicates that neural conditions in the brain are favorable for attentive effort, good performance, and the like. From the EEG pattern we cannot specify what the neurons are actually doing; because in order to do this, one must have unit and multiple unit recording, which is impossible without surgery. (Animal studies employing multiple unit recording techniques will be described presently.) However, for this discussion of EMG gradients from human subjects, it will be sufficient to use the continuously activated EEG pattern as a rough index of neural conditions that are favorable for involvement in an activity requiring concentrated effort. This seems reasonable in view of the confirmations from interest ratings by subjects and tests of their performance.

We return now to the Alice and the Red Queen phenomenon: that is, the problem posed by the EMG gradient representing rising muscular activity over a period of time when quality of performance remains level (and the EEG remains the same). The diagram in Figure 5.3 suggests a possible solution to this problem. We assume facilitative activation (at some optimal level) by the neurons in the reticular core to be an essential condition for good performance. Now suppose that the neocortical neuronal circuits adapt to facilitatory bombardment (as central neurons are known to do). Then the cortical circuits would require more and more input from the reticular core over the period when the person was applying himself continuously to some task. Now look in the diagram at the descending reticulo-spinal tracts. It is clear from the discussion in Chapter III and from our knowledge of the reticular system that this part of the motor system is an integral part of the behavioral sequences (whether it be tracking, listening to a story, thinking, or whatever). Now if, as we have reason to believe, the muscles adapt less to continuous activation than do neurons in the cortical circuits, we have one possible explanation for the rising gradients. In the relative absence of adaptation by the muscles, the EMGs would reveal the progressively increasing input from the reticular core by progressively increasing contractions, which, of course, is what the EMG gradients are.

The reticular core is so strategically placed that, as might be expected, it participates in a wide variety of neurophysiological functions, which are beyond the scope of this book.

Through the mammalian series, the reticular core has changed less than most other parts of the brain. It should not be thought of as a homogeneous network, because it contains various differentiated nuclei (groups of cell bodies). Nevertheless, it is useful to consider its appearance of integrated function, especially with regard to its influence on behavior.

The reticular core appears to be ideally structured to develop the kind of "build-up" of neuronal activation that EMG gradients reflect. In the reticular core are millions of reentrant loops, which in their feedback potentialities, appear ideally suited for just this kind of rising function. In fact, one might wonder how the build-up could ever be stopped once it was underway. The answer to this problem seems to somehow involve the multiple inputs to the reticular core which compete for control of the reticular arrays. At the psychological level, these would appear to be the internal and external stimulating conditions that are responsible for bringing the tension down, and thus terminating the gradient.

NEUROPHYSIOLOGICAL EXPERIMENTS ON
THE RETICULAR CORE AND BEHAVIOR

Now we shall consider some important experiments with animals, in order to learn something about the effects of electrically stimulating the reticular core, and recording from it.

Experiments by Fuster and Uyeda

Figure 5.4 shows the apparatus that these neurophysiologists used to study the effects of reticular-formation stimulation on performance efficiency.

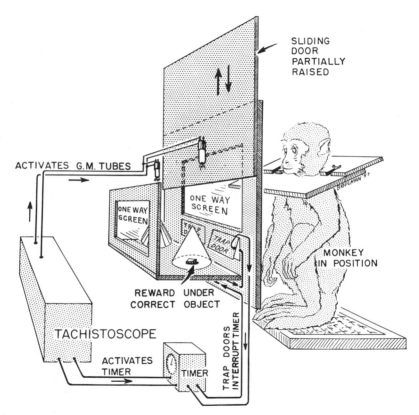

Figure 5.4 *Diagram of apparatus used by Fuster and Uyeda (1962) to study the effects of reticular-formation stimulation on performance efficiency of monkeys.* The monkey sits in a restraining box facing a one-way screen. On the other side of the screen are two objects, a cone and a 12-sided pyramid. Trial commences when experimenter lifts opaque screen. One second later a bell is sounded, followed two seconds later by a brief illumination of the object. Having viewed the two objects briefly, the monkey now puts his hands through the trap doors to reach the objects. He is taught to raise the cone (not the pyramid) and is rewarded, each time, by finding a small piece of diced apple under the cone. If he raises the pyramid, this is an error and he finds no apple. The time it took the monkey to raise the object is recorded by the timer. The objects are changed about from trial to trial randomly, so that the monkey learns it is the cone (and not merely position: right or left) to which he must attend. G.M. Tubes: Glow Modulator Tubes. (After Fuster & Uyeda, Facilitation of tachistoscopic performance by stimulation of midbrain tegmental points in the monkey. *Experimental Neurology*, 1962, *6*, 384–406. Reproduced by permission of Academic Press and the author.)

Fuster and Uyeda (1962) found that'there was an optimal level of reticular stimulation for best performance (accurate, fast reactions). Performance suffered when stimulation was higher than this optimal level. Stimulation of brain areas outside the reticular formation did not produce these effects. Therefore the brain stimulations were not merely signaling the monkey when to look.

Galin and Lacey (1972) in work with cats have confirmed the beneficial effects of reticular stimulation on reaction-time performance.

A possible objection to this experimental procedure is that brain stimulation is unnatural, and therefore that the results might not occur under more natural circumstances. Fortunately, there is an answer to this kind of criticism in Goodman's (1968) experiments.

Goodman's Experiments

Goodman trained thirsty rhesus monkeys to press a bar in front of them in order to receive a little water through a drinking tube. When a red light came on, the monkey was required to press the bar quickly; because if the light went out before he pressed, he received no water.

After training the monkeys, Goodman implanted electrodes in their midbrain reticular formations. These electrodes picked up the firing of a number of nerve cells and fed the signals into an amplifying and recording system. This is called *multiple-unit* recording. Figure 5.5 shows illustrations of recordings made during testing. Results confirmed the conclusions of Fuster and Uyeda (1962). There is a level of reticular-neuron activity that is optimal for performance. Above and below this optimal level, performance is relatively poor.

The kind of reticular activity most favorable for efficient performance was steady firing at a moderate level just prior to stimulation. Sudden change in activity of the reticular neurons at the time of stimulation was unfavorable for performance. Top tracings in Figure 5.5 illustrate this kind of unfavorable condition.

Goodman's observations are remarkable for their extreme consistency. He found that all short reaction times (less than 300 milliseconds) were preceded by reticular activity in the moderate (66–73 percent) range. In other words, moderate reticular activity was a *necessary* condition for a short reaction time.

It is clearly an oversimplification to suppose that activation from the reticular core is important only because of its firing into the neocortex. It seems likely that the downward activation through the motor pathways that descend to the spinal cord is just as important for performance. As a matter of fact, Goodman observed that the best recording sites for his

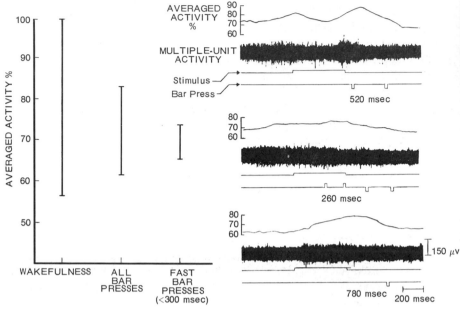

Figure 5.5 *Goodman's experiment showing that the necessary condition for fast reaction time is a moderate amount of neural activity in the reticular system.* When neural activity is either above or below this optimal amount, performance suffers. The middle set of tracings on the right side are typical of those accompanying a fast reaction, which in this case was 260 thousandths of a second (260 milliseconds). The broader the jagged black band and the more evident the multiple spikes, the greater the amount of multineuronal firing. These records are photographs taken from an oscilloscope. The thin line above each oscilloscope tracing is a continuous averaging of the multiple-unit activity (taking both frequency of spiking and height of spikes into account). Percentage values opposite this line represent percent of maximal multiple-unit activity, with 100 percent being the amount of neural activity observed immediately after the monkey had been startled by a loud sound. Necessary condition for short reaction time (less than 300 milliseconds) was a multineuronal activity average between 66 and 73 percent. In middle tracings (associated with fast reaction time) the averaged multiple-unit activity at onset of visual stimulus was between 66 and 73 percent. Lower tracings illustrate percent lower than 66 percent at stimulus onset and long reaction time. Upper tracings illustrate percent higher than 73 percent and long reaction time again. Brackets to left of tracings show (a) the optimal range of percentages for fast reaction times (66–73 percent), (b) range for all bar-presses, including slow reaction times, and (c) the total waking range, from quiet rest with eyes open to the high level of multineuronal activity produced by startling the monkey. (After Goodman, Visuo-motor reaction times and brain stem multiple-unit activity. *Experimental Neurology*, 1968, *22*, 367–378. Reproduced by permission of Academic Press and the author.)

experiments were those that, during operation, showed increased neuronal activity when the animal moved slightly as the anesthesia lightened.

The effects of reticular activity on other kinds of performance have been observed. In an earlier experiment, Goodman observed that cats ran faster along a runway when stimulated in the reticular formation; and this observation was confirmed by Sterman and Fairchild (1966) who observed that hungry cats ran faster toward food when stimulated in the reticular formation. There were no signs of pain with stimulation, only improved running performance.

Nakajima (1964) used moderate chemical excitation of the reticular formation to make hungry rats press faster on a bar for food pellets. When he increased chemical excitation beyond this moderate amount, the rats reduced their bar-pressing. In other words, he showed once again that moderate activation of the reticular system improved performance, and that too strong an activation made performance worse. In thorough control experiments, he showed that the effects were specific to the reticular system, and also that poor performance with overstimulation was not due to gross motor disturbances.

These neurophysiological data on the reticular system are extremely provocative in relation to problems under consideration in this chapter. Quite obviously they seem to run parallel to some of the key behavioral observations. The two sets of observations appear to be heading toward meaningful correlations although, of course, much further research is needed before we can begin to state these correlations in detail. At least we may formulate questions (state hypotheses) to guide future research.

It should be useful at this point to return to a consideration of some additional psychophysiological research.

PSYCHOPHYSIOLOGICAL RESEARCH ON BOREDOM AND OTHER DETRACTORS FROM GOOD PERFORMANCE

Boredom: Falling Physiological Levels and Declining Performance

When a person begins to perform a task (as subject) in a psychological laboratory, the novelty of the situation is stimulating. However, if the session is long and the task somewhat repetitive and boring, interest naturally wanes. In other words, motivation declines. What happens to performance and to physiological levels? There are some data on this question from recent experiments.

Davies and Krkovic (1965) gave college students a "vigilance" task to work on for a 90-minute period. Using a tape recorder, they presented a series of digits (1–9) in random order at the rate of one per second. The subject was told to listen for a series of three odd digits (for example, 5-1-7), and whenever he detected such a series, to press a key. There were only thirty-six such 3-digit series in the entire 90-minute period, so that minutes would go by with nothing to signal. (Digit sequences to be signaled were spaced irregularly: as brief as 21 seconds, and as long as 6½ minutes.)

The experimenters recorded electroencephalograms (EEGs) and palmar conductance (mainly a measure of sweating) throughout the 90 minutes. Figure 5.6 presents the results. The falling curves, which follow a remarkably similar time course, reflect progressive decline in motivation.

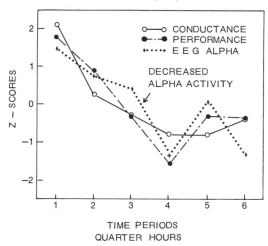

Figure 5.6 *Declining efficiency in a vigilance task, with accompanying progressive downward shifts in physiological levels.* Vigilance scores, levels of palmar conductance (chiefly a measure of sweating), and levels of EEG alpha activity (that is, in the EEG frequency range close to 10 waves per second) are shown. Scores for averaged values have been converted to Z scores to make comparisons easier. Curves show that as efficiency on the task declined during the session, there were corresponding downward shifts in the physiological measures. Level of palmar sweating progressed downward as did amplitude of EEG alpha. The large fall in palmar sweating is like that which is generally observed when alertness is decreasing. The EEG alpha change is like that commonly observed in persons drifting toward drowsiness. Note the remarkable agreement between curves. (After Davies & Krkovic, Skin-conductance, alpha-activity, and vigilance. *American Journal of Psychology*, 1965, *78*, 304–306.)

Some data from our laboratory (Malmo, 1966) confirm and extend these experimental findings. In our experiments, a group of forty-two male subjects tracked. Comparing performance scores and physiological measures from early in the session with those from later in the same session, we found significant differences in the averages. Performance declined late in the session and so did the physiological levels. Heart rate and breathing rate were lower, and palmar sweating was less. In addition, muscle tension (EMG) level, recorded from the left leg, was significantly lower later in the session than earlier.

The encouragement (incentive) provided by the experimenter is as strong toward the end as it was at the beginning of a long session in the laboratory. However, long exposure to the experimental situation has its own decremental effect, which is observable in relatively impaired performance and in lowered physiological levels.

This kind of efficiency loss is just opposite to the kind described at the beginning of this chapter, where overwhelming demands of emergency situations impaired performance. However, it can be just as disastrous when, for example, a driver becomes inattentive on a fast highway. Monotonous stimulation may well have a damping effect on the reticular system and, if so, this is a further instance of danger inherent in a "primordial" brain mechanism. Monotony of sensory stimulation may be a safety signal in primitive settings, but obviously not on the highway or in other mechanized settings.

Effects of Noise on Performance

The results of experiments with noise are interesting, and somewhat unexpected on common-sense grounds. However, they appear meaningful in relation to our discussion of reticular-system activity and performance. The effects of noise on performance depend on whether incentive is high or low.

Psychologists at the Applied Psychology Research Unit in Cambridge, England, found that noise reduced efficiency *only* when the men were working under high incentive, and not if they were relatively bored and unmotivated (see Hockey, 1969). With low-incentive boring tasks, better work was obtained under noisy than under quiet conditions. Clearly, the factors of background noise and incentive interacted to impair performance when incentive was high and to improve it when incentive was low.

It seems a reasonable guess that a brain mechanism like the reticular system could be involved in this interaction. Recall that Goodman used a sudden loud sound to drive reticular activity up to a high level (see Figure 5.5 and see the ascending sensory pathways to the reticular core represented in Figure 5.3). It is known that less intense auditory stimulation also increases the firing rate of certain neurons in the reticular core. Therefore, if incentive conditions also have an activating effect on neurons in the reticular core, the possibility of combined effects of noise and incentive is obvious. Again, these suggestions are to be regarded as questions for further research.

In order to communicate the ideas in this chapter, we have had to simplify matters. The reader must bear this in mind. For instance, we have spoken of the reticular system. The reader must realize that the neural structures involved are highly diversified, and that there are numerous connections with other parts of the brain. This is indicated in Figure 5.3, but the connections are much more complicated. It is encouraging, nonetheless, that so much progress has been made. Future research obviously has great promise.

On the behavioral side, too, we may be in danger of leaving the reader with an oversimplified notion about relations between efficiency and motivation. In order to correct any such impression, it will be useful to describe one more experiment from our laboratory. This is a companion experiment to the one on motivational lag (that is, boredom) developing late in the session.

With the same group of subjects, we were able to produce approximately the same drop in efficiency, without affecting physiological levels (see Malmo, 1966). Tracking, guided by sound, was done in precisely the same way as before. There was only one difference in procedure: the experimenter told the tracker that later in the trial he would have to shift to a more difficult task (double tracking).

Each subject had been trained earlier to engage in double tracking. While turning the hand-knob, tracking to auditory (tone) signals, he simultaneously operated a foot pedal like an automobile accelerator. Operation of the foot pedal was guided by two vibrators, one attached on the left, and the other on the right side of his chest. Except for the direction of motion (vertical, down to the floor and then up again, instead of rotary), the guidance (feedback) to the subject was the same in principle for this foot tracking as it was for hand tracking.

On some trials, the subject was told that he would not have to shift to double tracking. Average performance on these trials was significantly better than on the trials where the person was told that he must shift later to double tracking.

The loss of efficiency, as mentioned, was about the same with this "mental hazard" (expectancy) as it was with the "boredom" effect previously described. But again the two kinds of impairment were dissimilar physiologically. Expecting to have to shift over to double tracking reduced tracking efficiency but it had none of the effects on physiological levels that were observed in other kinds of impairment. (A wide variety of physiological measures failed to show even one significant change associated with this impairment.)

This negative finding places the impairment in a different category from some of the others that we have been discussing. It is an intriguing kind of impairment, incidentally, because what the person must do in both conditions is precisely the same: keep his attention on hand tracking and make a good score. The person gained no advantage from thinking about the double tracking before it commenced. But apparently the inability of the person to suppress the thoughts of what was coming interfered significantly with the task at hand. Note that the lack of change in physiological levels indicates that there was no change in effort or in motivation to do well.

We may throw some light on these perplexing findings by referring once again to the Goodman experiment on multiple-unit recording from the reticular system. Recall that an optimal level of reticular neuronal firing was a *necessary* condition for efficient performance. Now we may add his observation that it was not a *sufficient* condition. Never was there a fast reaction time when reticular activity was outside the moderate range. However, reticular activity could be within the moderate range, and the monkey might still have a *long* reaction time, if his attention was distracted by something extraneous to the environment, such as a door being opened.

SUMMARY

A well-coordinated, completely appropriate response depends on a highly complex sequence of events in the brain. From the neurophysiological point of view there are two aspects of this complex process. First, there is a *phasic* aspect, which involves the precise timing and sequential ordering of the different neural components of the act being performed. Second, there is a *tonic* aspect, which involves continuous facilitation of the phasic sequence by a tonic activating neural mechanism.

In this chapter we have been considering the neuropsychological significance of tonic background activity. We concluded that there is an optimal level of this background neural activity (referred to as level of "arousal" or "activation"). When phasic acts are carried out under conditions of optimal arousal, they are better coordinated and more efficient than when they are carried out under conditions of lower or higher arousal levels. Recent neuropsychological research, Goodman's in particular, has demonstrated the role of the reticular core of the brain stem in generating supportive tonic background neural activity for phasic acts.

Stennett's data from recordings of EMG and autonomic functions provide psychophysiological evidence for the validity of the principle of an optimal "arousal" level in relation to performance level. In the psychophysiological approach to the problem of "arousal," the unique importance of EMG gradients (described first in Chapter III) is clear; and it is reasonable to suppose that neural activity in the reticular core of the brain stem is largely responsible for this progressively rising background level of tonic muscular contractions.

Research reviewed in this chapter also showed how performance suffers when background arousal level is too low. These experimental findings are significant in relation to research on boredom, which revealed some interesting interactions. For instance, background noise actually helps performance when the subject's arousal level is low (that is, when bored), but the same noise hinders performance when his arousal level is high. This finding is interesting in relation to the fact that neural activity in part of the reticular core may be driven up by presenting loud sounds to the animal.

Finally, caution is important in order that these remarkably concordant relations do not lead us, in our enthusiasm, to overlook some of the complexities. For instance, it is possible to manipulate performance level by means other than varying involvement or other arousal factors. This was shown in the divided attention experiment. In this experiment, the instructions were designed to keep involvement and other arousal factors at the same level for both conditions. That these arousal factors were in fact equated under the two conditions was indicated by the absence of any significant differences in levels of physiological arousal from condition to condition. Recall that the subject's task was precisely the same in both conditions, the only difference being that of *expecting* to have to shift later to a more difficult task in the divided attention condition. This expectancy turned out to have an impairing effect on performance.

These puzzling findings are challenging. What seems most clear is that the conditions are sufficiently different from the other experiments in which positive physiological results *were* obtained to make it unreasonable to use these findings to discount the demonstrated relations between physiological arousal level and performance. The challenge is to discover what *divided attention* is, and to learn more about its effects on performance.

Returning to the problem of involvement, the fact that a subject performs at a higher level after listening to instructions designed to increase his involvement in performing the task indicates that the instructions were effective in activating a source of internal "push." This push reflects the operation of a complex, high-level kind of need. What it is in the brain that is activated in order to mediate this kind of need is unknown. However, there is information concerning brain mechanisms related to more primitive needs, such as the need for water, a topic that we shall consider in the next chapter.

In working toward the understanding of a need system in neural terms, it is a distinct advantage if one can discover a central sensor that detects and signals the need. If a central sensing mechanism can be discovered, one has a point of origin from which to work in going about the job of learning more and more about the system.

Fortunately, there are some recent neuropsychological experiments which strongly encourage the belief that the central sensors (receptors) for cellular dehydration thirst have been found. The next chapter will review some of these experiments in considering problems related to the innate need for water. In addition, certain "acquired needs" (for drugs) will be considered in a similar context.

REFERENCES

Broadbent, D. E. How noise affects work. *New Society*, 1966, March 3 number, 12–14.

Broadhurst, P. L. Emotionality and the Yerkes-Dodson law. *Journal of Experimental Psychology*, 1957, *54*, 345–352.

Caldwell, J. M., Ranson, S. W., & Sacks, J. G. Group panic and other mass disruptive reactions. *United States Armed Forces Medical Journal*, 1951, *2*, 541–567.

Davies, D. R., & Krkovic, A. Skin-conductance, alpha-activity, and vigilance. *American Journal of Psychology*, 1965, *78*, 304–306.

Ellison, G. D., Humphrey, G. L., & Feeney, D. M. Some electrophysiological correlates of classical and instrumental behavior. *Journal of Comparative and Physiological Psychology*, 1968, *66*, 340–348.

Fuster, J. M., & Uyeda, A. A. Facilitation of tachistoscopic performance by stimulation of midbrain tegmental points in the monkey. *Experimental Neurology*, 1962, *6*, 384–406.

Galin, D., & Lacey, J. I. Reaction time and heart rate response pattern: Effects of reticular stimulation in cats. *Physiology and Behavior*, 1972, *8*, 729–739.

Goodman, S. J. Visuo-motor reaction times and brain stem multiple-unit activity. *Experimental Neurology*, 1968, *22*, 367–378.

Hockey, R. Noise and efficiency: The visual task. *New Scientist*, 1969, 244–246.

Malmo, R. B. Finger-sweat prints in the differentiation of low and high incentive. *Psychophysiology*, 1965, *1*, 231–240.

Malmo, R. B. Cognitive factors in impairment: A neuropsychological study of divided set. *Journal of Experimental Psychology*, 1966, *71*, 184–189.

Marshall, S. L. A. *Men against fire*. New York: William Morrow, 1947.

Moruzzi, G., & Magoun, H. W. Brain stem reticular formation and activation of the EEG. *Electroencephalography and Clinical Neurophysiology*, 1949, *1*, 455–473.

Nakajima, S. Effects of chemical injection into the reticular formation of rats. *Journal of Comparative and Physiological Psychology*, 1964, *58*, 10–15.

Olds, J. The central nervous system and the reinforcement of behavior. *American Psychologist*, 1969, *24*, 114–132.

Starzl, T. E., Taylor, C. W., & Magoun, H. W. Collateral afferent excitation of reticular formation of brain stem. *Journal of Neurophysiology*, 1951, *14*, 479–496.

Stennett, R. G. The relationship of performance level to level of arousal. *Journal of Experimental Psychology*, 1957, *54*, 54–61.

Sterman, M. B., & Fairchild, M. D. Modification of locomotor performance by reticular formation and basal forebrain stimulation in the cat: Evidence for reciprocal systems. *Brain Research*, 1966, *2*, 205–217.

Tyhurst, J. S. Individual reactions to community disaster. The natural history of psychiatric phenomena. *American Journal of Psychiatry*, 1951, *107*, 764–769.

VI

On Needs: Inborn and Acquired

PICTURE EIGHT MEN stranded without food or drinking water, sitting in three rubber life rafts, which they had inflated after their plane had crashed into the Pacific Ocean. This is the situation that Eddie Rickenbacker and his companions found themselves in during World War II. The following are some quotations from his story, reproduced in part in Wolf (1958).

> Now, memories of food and drink began to haunt us. . . .
>
> Reynolds talked about how much soda pop he was going to drink the rest of his life. Cherry couldn't think about anything but chocolate ice cream. As I listened to the thirsty talk between the rafts, my own mind slowly filled with visions of chocolate malted milk. I could actually taste it, to the point where my tongue worked convulsively. The strange part is that I hadn't had a chocolate malted milk in nearly 25 years.
>
> . . . when I was dozing with my hat pulled down over my eyes, a gull appeared from nowhere and landed on my hat.
>
> I don't remember how it happened or how I knew he was there. But I knew it instantly, and I knew that if I missed this one, I'd never find another to sit on my hat. I reached up for him with my right hand— gradually. The whole Pacific seemed to be shaking from the agitation in my body, but I could tell he was still there from the hungry, famished, almost insane eyes in the other rafts. Slowly and surely my hand got up

there; I didn't clutch, but just closed my fingers, sensing his nearness, then closing my fingers hard.

I wrung his neck, defeathered him, carved up the body, divided the meat into equal shares, holding back only the intestines for bait. Even the bones were chewed and swallowed. No one hesitated because the meat was raw and stringy and fishy. It tasted fine. After Cherry had finished his piece, I baited a hook and passed it over to him. The hook, weighted with Whittaker's ring, had hardly got wet before a small mackerel hit it, and was jerked into the raft. I dropped the other line, with the same miraculous result, except that mine was a small sea bass.

All this food in the space of a few minutes bolstered us beyond words. We ate one of the fish before dark, put the other aside for the next day. Even the craving for water seemed to abate, perhaps from chewing the cool, wet flesh while grinding the bones to a pulp (pp. 435–436).[1]

Under ordinary circumstances, of course, food and water are readily available. Consequently we generally experience only mild thirst and pleasant appetite for food. But under conditions of deprivation, of the kind Rickenbacker described, thirst and hunger become powerful drives indeed and, of course, have great survival value in signaling need for water and food.

Need for water is especially critical since death from lack of water occurs sooner than death from starvation. Because of its extraordinary biological significance, thirst is chosen for our present discussion of innate need. The initial problem for the neuropsychologist is to find out how depletion of water in tissues is detected. It was natural for early theories about thirst to consider dryness of the mouth to be the point of origin in the chain of neurophysiological events mediating thirst and water-seeking behavior. This concept goes back to the philosopher Descartes and it persisted as a working hypothesis as late as 1929, in the Harvard laboratory of the great physiologist Walter B. Cannon. However, the experimental work generated by this hypothesis invalidated the concept. For instance, making dogs' throats dry by removing their salivary glands failed to make the dogs drink more water.

Research has now made it clear that many of the receptors signaling need for water are located in the brain itself. Because of their location within the central nervous system, they are called *central* receptors. We proceed now to review the highlights of our knowledge about the neuropsychology of thirst.

[1] From *Seven Came Through* by E. V. Rickenbacker. New York: Doubleday & Company, Inc. Copyright 1943. Reprinted by permission.

MECHANISMS FOR PROTECTION OF THE BODY
AGAINST EXCESSIVE LOSS OF WATER

About 60 percent of the total body weight of the human adult is water. Water in the cells accounts for about 40 percent of the total body weight. The other 20 percent is in the fluids outside the cells (*extracellular*

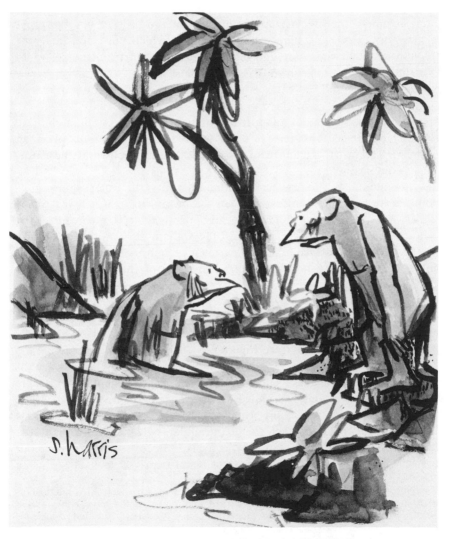

"Take it from me and come back. The future is definitely on land." (From *American Scientist*, 1971, *59*, 415. Reprinted by permission of cartoonist Sidney Harris.)

fluids). The latter is referred to as the *extracellular compartment* and the former as the *cellular compartment*.

Recent research has shown that there are at least two factors determining thirst: (a) cellular dehydration thirst, and (b) extracellular dehydration thirst.

It has been said that we mammals carry the sea about with us as we move on land, and to a certain extent this is indeed true. Considering that about 60 percent of our body weight is water, it is easy to see that water is vital to the life-sustaining functions of the cells in our body. As we move about on land our bodies lose water, which must constantly be replenished. Otherwise more and more water is drawn from the cells into the extracellular compartment. As we shall see, the exchange of water between the cells and the extracellular compartment is of key importance in the neuropsychology of thirst.

With the sea theme in mind, it is intriguing that salt (sodium chloride or NaCl) dissolved in water (referred to as a *saline solution*) plays an important role in the exchange of water between the cells and the extracellular compartment.

In a mammal who has had continuous access to water, and consequently is in a normally hydrated state, the percent of NaCl in the extracellular and intracellular fluids is nearly identical at 0.9 percent. Now when the animal is deprived of water, the sodium chloride concentration is increased in the extracellular compartment, while the intracellular NaCl concentration remains at 0.9 percent. The cause of this disequilibrium is the cell membrane, which blocks the passage of the NaCl molecule into the cell.

The higher concentration of NaCl outside than inside the cell increases the osmotic pressure such that water is forced out of the cells into the extracellular fluids (see Figure 6.1). Note that the cell membrane allows water molecules to pass through, while blocking the passage of sodium chloride molecules. This kind of membrane, which is permeable to certain molecules only, is called *semipermeable*. A 0.9 percent NaCl solution is *isotonic*, while any NaCl concentration higher than this is called *hypertonic*. The higher the extracellular NaCl concentration, the greater the flow of water out of the cells.[2] Since sea water is about 3 percent NaCl it is understandable that water-deprived men at sea (like

---

[2] *Osmosis* means the passage of a solvent through a membrane from a dilute solution to a more concentrated one. Molecules of the solute on the more concentrated side of the membrane bombard the membrane more frequently on that side. This means that they exert a greater fraction of the total pressure. For our purposes, the concentration of the sodium chloride solution may be considered as commensurate with *osmolarity*, which is the effect of the given concentration upon *osmotic pressure*. The higher the concentration of the NaCl solution the greater is its osmolarity and the greater the increase in osmotic pressure.

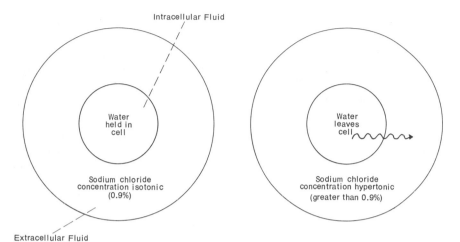

Figure 6.1 *Intracellular and extracellular fluids.* Water is drawn from cells into extracellular fluids when the body has lost water. Appreciable loss of water from the body increases concentration of sodium chloride or NaCl (ordinary "table salt") in extracellular fluids. Increased extracellular sodium concentration draws water from cells by *osmotic pressure.* Loss of water from the body can be simulated by injections of a salt solution that is more concentrated than that found in the normal hydrated condition. A salt solution that is this concentrated is called *hypertonic*; that found in normal hydrated condition (0.9 percent NaCl) is called *isotonic.*

Rickenbacker and his companions, but less knowledgeable) have hastened their deaths by drinking sea water. The strongly hypertonic sea water rapidly reduces the water content of the cells to lethal limits.

Osmoreceptors: Brain Cells that Signal Loss of Water

When the mammal has been deprived of water, all body cells lose water to the hypertonic extracellular compartment. This includes cells in the brain (neurons). However, only certain neurons are specialized to *sense* the extracellular hypertonicity and to signal it by changing their rates of firing (usually in the direction of increased firing rate). Because of their sensory function and because of their location in the central nervous system, these cells are called *central receptors.* E. B. Verney named them *osmoreceptors* because they are specialized to sense changes in the osmotic pressure of the extracellular fluids.

It is a credit to Verney's imagination that he inferred the existence of osmoreceptors from some brilliant observations in his physiological laboratory. Verney's experiments were done prior to the development of brain-recording techniques that enable the neurophysiologist to observe the firing rate of single neurons.

Recording from Osmoreceptors   Osmoreceptors are neurons that change their firing rates (usually in the direction of a faster rate) when the surrounding extracellular fluids become hypertonic. The most extensive research on osmoreceptors has been done in J. N. Hayward's laboratory at the University of California in Los Angeles.

Although Hayward's elegant apparatus is fairly elaborate, the basic methodology of single-neuron recording technique is easy to grasp. The end of the tungsten wire microelectrode is pointed by means of electrolytical etching to a tip diameter of one micrometer (one millionth of a meter) or less. A microscope is used to determine the precise diameter

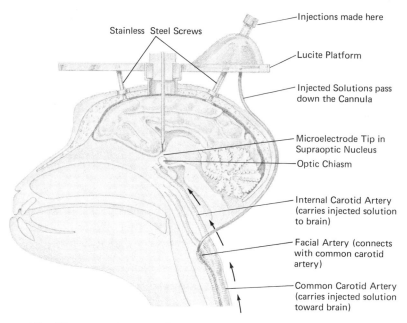

Figure 6.2   *Diagrammatic view of apparatus for recording from osmoreceptors in the monkey's brain while injecting hypertonic saline solution into carotid artery (carrying blood supply to the brain).*   Microelectrode picks up discharges from single cell in supraoptic nucleus of hypothalamus (nucleus gets its name from its location, lying as it does just above the optic chiasm, part of the visual system). Through surgery on the monkey's neck, a cannula (tube for carrying saline solution) is placed into the facial artery, which connects with the common carotid artery. The other end of the cannula is led underneath the skin and brought out to the dome-shaped structure shown at top right. Inside this structure, the open end of the cannula is fitted over a hypodermic needle, which is attached to a cap that is designed to receive injections. By means of a calibrated syringe, injections are made through this cap. Not shown in the diagram is a device for accurately placing and holding the electrode in the supraoptic nucleus. All surgery was done with monkeys under anesthesia. Recordings were made later when animals had recovered from surgery and were awake. Monkeys showed no signs of anxiety or discomfort during recording. (After Hayward & Vincent, Osmosensitive single neurones in the hypothalamus of unanaesthetized monkeys. *Journal of Physiology*, 1970, *210*, 947–972.)

of the tip. A stereotaxic instrument is used to guide the placement of the electrode in the brain of the anesthetized animal.

Figure 6.2 shows the position of the microelectrode tip in one of the monkeys used by Hayward and Vincent. Note that the tip is located in brain tissue that is just above the optic chiasm (the crossing point of visual fibers coming from the eye). The nucleus (that is, population of neurons) in which the electrode tip rests is called the *supraoptic nucleus* because of its location just above these optic fibers. The microelectrode tip is resting next to the cell membrane of an osmoreceptor in the supraoptic nucleus. When the osmoreceptor fires, there is an accompanying distinct voltage change, which is picked up by the electrode and observed as a spikelike deflection on a cathode ray oscilloscope screen. The lower part of Figure 6.3 shows three trains of spikes, which represent three different

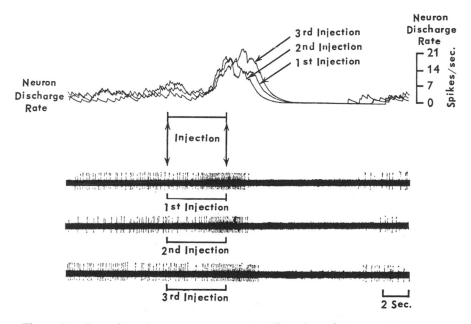

Figure 6.3 *Recordings from an osmoreceptor.* They show three separate responses, each to intracarotid injection of saline solution (see Figure 6.2). The three injections were spaced two minutes apart. Three tracings in lower part of figure show firing of cell as photographically recorded from an oscilloscope. Each spike represents one discharge or firing of the brain cell. Soon after saline injection, the firing rate increased and then subsided. These cells are sensitive to small injections of hypertonic sodium chloride into the carotid artery, but show little or no response to arousing sensory stimuli (for example, sounds or touches). Upper tracings are from integrating device that writes out the graph: the higher the line on the graph, the greater the rate of neuron discharge. Note again in these graphs the responses of the neuron to injections. (After Hayward & Vincent, Osmosensitive single neurones in the hypothalamus of unanaesthetized monkeys. *Journal of Physiology,* 1970, *210,* 947–972.)

periods of observing the activity of the same osmoreceptor. Note how the rate of firing increased within the brief time period indicated by the brackets. During the period indicated by the brackets, the extracellular fluids surrounding the osmoreceptor were made hypertonic.

In order to make the extracellular fluids hypertonic, the experimenter injects a small amount of hypertonic (that is, greater than 0.9 percent) NaCl (saline) solution into the carotid artery, which supplies blood to the brain (see Figure 6.2). We should add that the greater the hypertonicity (for example, the higher the NaCl concentration), the stronger the reaction of the osmoreceptor.

Thus far, we have seen how the osmoreceptors respond to increased hypertonicity of their extracellular environment. Next, we consider the effects of this increased firing rate on the animal's bodily functions. This story is told in Figure 6.4. When the osmoreceptors in the supraoptic nucleus fire, they send impulses through their axons (long fibers attached to nerve cells) to the posterior (back) part of the pituitary gland, which releases a hormone into the blood stream. This hormone has an anti-diuretic effect (that is, the effect of shutting off or greatly reducing urine output), thus conserving water for the body. Urine when passed has a lower water content and hence is more concentrated than it normally is. The hormone acts on the kidney tubules, promoting their reabsorption

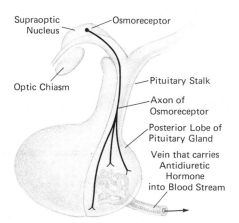

Supraoptic
Nucleus
Osmoreceptor
Optic Chiasm
Pituitary Stalk
Axon of
Osmoreceptor
Posterior Lobe of
Pituitary Gland
Vein that carries
Antidiuretic
Hormone
into Blood Stream

Figure 6.4 *Diagram illustrating the role of the supraoptic nucleus and the posterior pituitary gland in the antidiuretic reflex, which opposes or prevents excretion of urine.* Osmoreceptors in the supraoptic nucleus discharge into the posterior (back) part of the pituitary gland, causing release of antidiuretic hormone into the blood stream. When the antidiuretic hormone reaches the kidneys, it promotes reabsorption of water by the kidney tubules, thus conserving water for the body. See Figures 6.2 and 6.3 and text for explanation of osmoreceptors. Supraoptic nucleus is main location of osmoreceptors for the antidiuretic reflex.

of water. Current research indicates that at least some of the osmoreceptors are *neurosecretory* (that is, capable of secreting the antidiuretic hormone).

Projection of the osmoreceptor's axonal terminals into the posterior pituitary can be proved by electrically stimulating the axon terminal in the posterior pituitary and observing the firing of the osmoreceptor cell. This kind of stimulation is called *antidromic* because it causes the axon to conduct in the direction that is opposite to the normal direction, which is always from the nerve cell outward along the axon.

Proof that these brain cells are truly osmoreceptors, and not merely second-order cells being fired by other neurons, has come from experiments in which these brain cells in the supraoptic nucleus have been surgically separated from adjacent neural tissue. It has also been possible to fire these cells directly by means of microinjections of minute quantities of mildly hypertonic NaCl solutions. Tiny cannulas (tubes for saline to pass through) are implanted in the brain so that a minute quantity of saline can be injected directly onto the circumscribed neural area.

The antidiuretic reflex is obviously useful for survival of the mammal when deprived of water. A rat can live for 2 to 3 weeks without water; but for survival beyond this period, water-seeking, water-ingesting neural mechanisms must operate. What is known about them?

To begin with, these behavioral mechanisms have their own osmoreceptors, which lie outside the supraoptic nucleus. In the rat (Blass & Epstein, 1971) and rabbit (Peck & Novin, 1971) osmoreceptors have been found in the *preoptic* nucleus, so named because it is located in front of the optic chiasm (and so in front of the supraoptic nucleus). Lesions in the lateral preoptic nuclei were found to interfere with drinking, and microinjections of hypertonic solutions into the lateral preoptic area regularly initiated drinking, whereas the same injections elsewhere in the brain (including the supraoptic nucleus) failed to do so.

Figure 6.5 shows the activating effect of an injection of hypertonic NaCl on a cell in a rat's lateral preoptic area. In recording this change in the firing rate of the cell, we followed the basic procedures that were employed in Hayward's laboratory (see Figure 6.2 and 6.3). Our rats were anesthetized with urethane, which has relatively little effect on the cell's firing activity. The firing pattern is of the "burster" variety, which has also been observed in Hayward's laboratory. In our laboratory we have observed more neuronal activity in the lateral than in the medial preoptic area following intracarotid hypertonic saline injection. This parallels the findings of Blass and Epstein who have observed greater interference with drinking from lesions placed in the lateral than from those placed in the medial preoptic area.

The evidence favors the conclusion that the lateral preoptic area

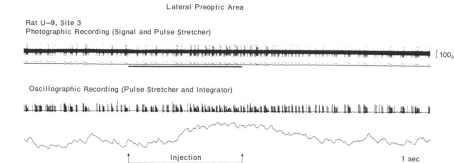

Figure 6.5 *Cell from rat's lateral preoptic nucleus, firing in "burster" pattern.* It increases its rate of firing in response to injection of hypertonic saline into the carotid artery. Top line: photograph taken from oscilloscope. Middle line: oscillographic ink recording of neuron's firing. (Section of oscillograph trace, duplicating information from oscilloscope.) Bottom line: trace of integrator recorder showing the reactions. (From Malmo & Mundl, Osmosensitive neurons in the rat's preoptic area: Medial-lateral comparison. *Journal of Comparative and Physiological Psychology*, in press.)

contains osmoreceptors for a major component of thirst, which is called *cellular dehydration thirst.* The distinctive feature of cellular dehydration thirst is hypertonicity of extracellular fluids with consequent loss of water by the cells. Recently, Fitzsimons (1972) has been responsible for calling attention to the importance of another component of the total thirst mechanism, that of *extracellular dehydration* thirst (or hypovolemia), which is caused by a reduction in the volume of extracellular fluids. During hemorrhage, for example, the volume of fluids in the extracellular compartment is suddenly reduced appreciably without any immediate change in hypertonicity. Such a condition, which is thirst-producing, is associated with increased quantities of certain hormones in the blood (renin, angiotensin I, and angiotensin II). Angiotensin II, especially, is now thought to play a key role in hypovolemic thirst. However, in contrast with the situation in *intra*cellular dehydration thirst, the receptors for *extra*cellular dehydration thirst are as yet unknown. No cells corresponding to the osmoreceptors have been discovered for hypovolemia.

Osmoreceptors and the receptors for hypovolemia (when they are known) provide points of origin in the neural system for thirst and water-related behavior.

The osmoreceptor's increased firing rate represents an internal *push* which, in interaction with external *pull* from the environment, instigates drinking behavior. The importance of this interaction can hardly be over-emphasized. We have observed 48-hour water-deprived rats (having lost 20 percent of their body weight) that fail to drink water placed directly under their noses in an observation box to which they had not become thoroughly habituated. The internal push was certainly there, but there was insufficient external pull to initiate drinking behavior. The converse is, of course, true: a water-sated rat in a familiar test box may fail to drink water because the internal push is missing. However, the quantity of water drunk by a laboratory rat is determined more by *external* factors than is generally recognized. For instance, recently it was reported that rats drank significantly more of their home-cage water when experimenters went in and out of the animal room frequently than when entrances into the room were relatively infrequent (Wright, 1972).

Proof that there are osmoreceptors is of considerable general importance for the psychology of needs. This proof gives concrete substance to a brain mechanism for internal push; and it encourages the hope that eventually some of the present candidates for central receptors for other needs (such as hunger) may also be substantiated.

ACQUIRED NEEDS

The concept of a central receptor as a mediator of internal push is also heuristic in approaching the problem of certain *acquired* needs (such as drug addictions) from the neuropsychological point of view.

Suppose we adopt the working hypothesis that the morphine addict in need of a "fix" has his internal push mediated by brain cells that act *in principle* like osmoreceptors. Instead of responding to hypertonicity of the extracellular fluids, we hypothesize that they respond to some other kind of chemical change in the extracellular fluids produced by deprivation of morphine.[3]

Weeks (1964) showed that rats can be made dependent on morphine by repeatedly injecting them with morphine over a period of time. Then when they were deprived of morphine, the rats would press a bar to inject themselves by means of an indwelling injection device. A plastic tube was passed under the skin from behind the ears to the front of the neck, where it was connected to a silicone-rubber cannula inserted into the rat's jugular vein. Rats addicted to morphine will also learn to drink bitter morphine solutions, which they normally reject (Stolerman & Kumar, 1970). From the morphine-dependent rat's behavior, it is obvious that he has acquired a new internal push (to apply the terminology that we have been using in connection with thirst).

Descriptions of the behavior of morphine-dependent chimpanzees

---

[3] The parallel between drug addiction and innate needs has been drawn by Hebb (1949), and by Skinner (1953).

(Spragg, 1940) impress one with the humanlike character of the behavior; but at the same time, one also sees the strong similarity between rat and chimpanzee in the way both developed drug dependence.

Figure 6.6 shows how Velt cooperated to receive a morphine injection. After some preliminary training, the chimpanzee accepted the injections when praised for being cooperative. Once the animal reached the stage where he readily accepted morphine injections, the injections

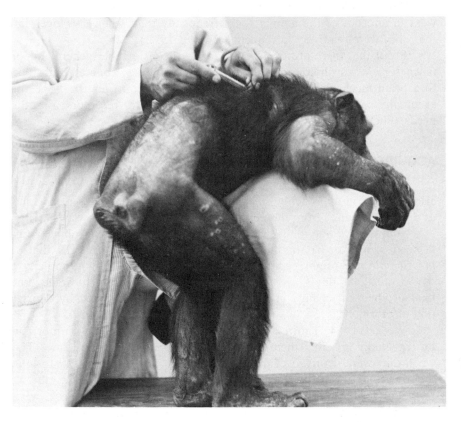

Figure 6.6 *Velt receiving morphine injection.* Spragg trained the chimpanzee to lean across his leg when he placed his foot up on the bench. Injection area is out of the chimpanzee's sight. Spragg began by training animals to tolerate mild scratching with an ordinary needle, giving them fruit as a reward for their cooperation. After experience, the chimpanzees tolerated scratching and pricking, even when quite vigorous; and later in training Spragg substituted a hypodermic needle for the ordinary needle and injected small amounts of nonnarcotic (saline) solution. Eventually, chimpanzees cooperated with only verbal approbation as reward (or none at all); and at this point morphine injections commenced. (From Spragg, Morphine addiction in chimpanzees. *Comparative Psychology Monographs*, 1940, *15*, (7, Whole No. 79). Copyright 1940 by the American Psychological Association, and reproduced by permission. Photo courtesy of Yerkes Regional Primate Research Center, Emory University.)

were kept up regularly, day after day. Eventually the chimpanzee learned to seek out the injection on his own initiative.

After learning, the chimpanzee showed eagerness to be taken from the living cage by the experimenter when doses were needed. He tugged at the leash, leading the experimenter toward and into the room in which injections were regularly given. The chimpanzee now showed eagerness and excitement when preparations were being made for the injection, no longer merely tolerating the injections, but cooperating eagerly in the injection procedure.

When a dose was needed, the animal clearly preferred morphine injection to food, even when he was very hungry. This he showed repeatedly by choosing a syringe-containing box (whereupon injection was given) in preference to a food-containing box. The addicted chimpanzee always showed obvious frustration when led away from the injection room and back to the living cage without having been given an injection.

Lyn, needing an injection, became excited when he saw Spragg at a distance approaching his cage. Spragg's observations showed that the chimpanzee's motor activation was specifically related to need for morphine, and not merely a general excitement associated with food or with a visit from Spragg. For example, Lyn was restless, and cried in the morning when Spragg came to his cage. This agitated behavior continued after breakfast, and only ceased *after* injection.

The foregoing descriptions provide clear examples of interactions between the two factors of internal push and external pull. We can only speculate about what structures in the brain might provide the push in morphine addiction.

Our working hypothesis is that there is a sensor resembling the osmoreceptor, which monitors the morphine level in the extracellular fluids. It is conceivable that certain brain cells, not already specialized for detecting dehydration or other such primary need states, may somehow undergo modification during the course of continuous morphine administration, thereby acquiring the properties of a central receptor. Actually, this possibility is open to experimental investigation. By means of microelectrode recording, one may search for brain cells that fire at a faster rate prior to a needed injection and reduce their rate of firing after injection. Therefore, this speculation has the merit of suggesting some experiments.

In considering what the physicochemical changes in the extracellular fluids could be, we have to realize that the nature of the cellular adaptation in states of drug dependence (and tolerance) is still an unsolved problem that presents a challenge to the physiologist and biochemist. Two kinds of theory about dependency may be distinguished. Both models postulate changes in the extracellular fluids that influence the firing rates of brain cells. According to one theory it is important for the drug to be on the neuron itself. According to the other theory (Jaffe & Sharpless, 1968), it is not the exposure of the neurons to the drug itself that is important, but the generalized blocking (or depressing) effect of the drug on the level of neural activity, which is followed by a rebound hyper-excitability. This increased excitation, on rebound, could be one of the sources of push in the person who has become drug-dependent.

Withdrawal Symptoms

Withdrawal symptoms differ from one addiction to another. Those observed by Spragg in his chimpanzees are commonly observed also in human morphine addicts. Spragg controlled the injections so that only mild withdrawal symptoms were produced. These were yawning (see Figure 6.7), running nose, drops of perspiration on the face, unusually large quantity of feces in the cage, and heightened irritability.

With longer withdrawal periods than Spragg imposed, more severe symptoms are produced in morphine addicts. As time without morphine goes on, the addict becomes increasingly more irritable, is frequently unable to eat or sleep, and shows increased severity of bodily symptoms: violent yawning, severe sneezing, and other signs resembling a bad cold. At this stage weakness may be pronounced; sweating, nausea and vomiting, intestinal spasm, and diarrhea can occur. Heart rate and blood pressure are sometimes abnormally high. These and other bodily changes can be dramatically reversed at any time by dosage with the drug.

While it is of course true that drug addicts dread the thought of having withdrawal symptoms, it would be oversimplifying matters to con-sider that avoidance of withdrawal symptoms is the addict's sole motivation in taking the drug.

A patient taking morphine under a physician's skillful care may go for months without experiencing withdrawal symptoms, and still look forward with pleasure to each injection. The injection itself is pleasurable to the human morphine user, and apparently Spragg's chimpanzees became calm after their injections, even prior to the physiological effects from the injection. There is probably some kind of *feedforward* mechanism oper-ating here.

An excellent example of a feedforward mechanism (though not drug related) is the following, which is taken from the work of Nicolaïdis (1964). It is a well-established fact that if persons are water-deprived and then placed in an overheated room the sweating that would occur in a normally hydrated person is greatly reduced in the dehydrated subject. In other words, the physiological mechanism for conservation of water

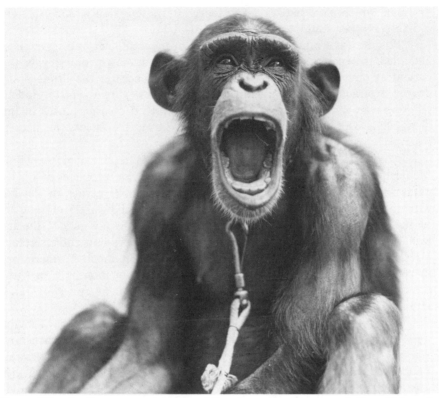

Figure 6.7   *A chimpanzee morphine addict, Lyn, showing one of his withdrawal symptoms: yawning.*   The mouth was usually held wide open for 3 or 4 seconds, then closed abruptly. (From Spragg, Morphine addiction in chimpanzees. *Comparative Psychology Monographs*, 1940, *15*, (7, Whole No. 79). Copyright 1940 by the American Psychological Association, and reproduced by permission. Photo courtesy of Yerkes Regional Primate Research Center, Emory University.)

is dominant over the one for thermoregulation. But a sweating response will occur in the dehydrated person 20 to 30 seconds following his ingestion of water in the hot room (that is, long before intestinal absorption of the water could have taken place). This anticipatory triggering of the sweating mechanism is a striking example of the feedforward principle. The same principle seems to be operating at the time of morphine injection, and feedforward is likely a more useful explanatory principle than feedback (from withdrawal symptoms) in accounting for the reinforcing effects of drug use.

Surely what makes a smoker take another cigarette has little or nothing to do with his fear of withdrawal symptoms per se; although it is true, of course, that some smokers who quit suddenly often do go through several weeks of distressing symptoms. The satisfaction from the first puff, which most smokers experience after a long nonsmoking interval is likely another example of feedforward.

Withdrawal symptoms are prominent in the treatment of drug addicts; and when the symptoms have entirely disappeared, most people regard the patient as having broken his "physical" dependence on the drug. Withdrawal treatments vary from sudden ("cold turkey") treatment to gradual tapering off over a period of 2 to 3 weeks, with decreasing doses of the drug and use of sedatives. If after the withdrawal treatment, the patient resumes his drug taking he is said to have *relapsed*.

According to the Canadian Commission of Inquiry into the Non-Medical Use of Drugs (1970) relapse is the major problem in opiate addiction. Employing the same kind of analysis used earlier in dealing with thirst, we can begin to see our way through the puzzle of relapse. In the first place, withdrawal techniques probably do not reduce the internal push factor to zero. It is well known that morphine addicts retain a residual "craving" for the drug after withdrawal treatment. Furthermore, there are reliable physiological deviations persisting for months after withdrawal procedures have been terminated (Wikler, 1968, p. 284; Jaffe, 1969, p. 352).

While withdrawal procedures seem to leave the internal push factor well above zero, still this factor is significantly reduced; so that now external pull factors become more important than before withdrawal. There is evidence of this from animal experiments. It has been shown that it is easier to readdict rats in the same environment where they were originally addicted than in a different environment (Thompson & Ostlund, 1965; Weeks & Collins, 1968). Stimuli in the familiar environment exert pull on the rat, probably by the same kind of interaction that occurs when a mildly thirsty rat is pulled in the direction of water by stimuli in a familiar watering place. (Note that environmental pull is always *selective*. Past experience determines this selectivity.)

In short, the readdicted rat is apparently a victim of internal push, from the residual internal alteration produced by the initial addictive procedures, interacting with the pull of *significant external* stimulation. Interestingly enough, animal experiments have conclusively shown that *some* internal push effect is required for an *external* stimulus to be at all effective in relation to the inborn needs of thirst and hunger. (See Valenstein's discussion of *incentive-motivation*, 1968, p. 68.)

There are enormous advantages in being able, in these animal studies, to strip away all the complex layers of human personality, so to speak, and to look at the core of the problems. Out of these animal studies come new ideas that can be applied to treatment of the human addict. For instance, it now seems evident that even after "complete withdrawal" the so-called postaddict is pulled toward readdiction by certain external stimuli in his environment because of the previous associations of these stimuli with drug-taking before "complete withdrawal," and because of the interaction of these stimuli with a residual internal state. Further researches on these external and internal factors, and on their interactions, are greatly needed.

This kind of analysis brings relapse into the same biological context with "physical" dependence. Looking at the problem in this way, it is no longer necessary to retain the mind-body dichotomy inherent in the distinction between "physical" and "psychological" dependence. The question is not whether this is a case of "physical" or "psychological" dependence; but instead: what are the significant interactions between *internal push* and *external pull* factors?

Working through these problems at the neuropsychological level provides a sound basis for dealing with social factors in addiction. Former drug takers must reorganize their conduct. This brings in the whole field of social motivation. Being partially freed from the grip of an acquired tissue need, the individual can be helped to reorganize the valuations of his own behavior, and also be influenced by the appropriate valuations from other persons of significance to him or her. The same things are true of alcoholics.

USE AND ABUSE OF ALCOHOL

A brief consideration of alcohol concludes this discussion of needs: inborn and acquired. Alcohol is especially interesting in relation to this topic because of the subtle mixtures of natural appetitive phenomena and the phenomena related to heavy drinking, dependency, and withdrawal symptoms (that is, the classical alcoholism syndrome).

There are results of alcohol abuse that stem from its intoxicating effects (e.g., impaired driving, overaggressive behavior), which have no counterpart in most medically supervised drug taking. The true parallel between drug addiction and alcoholism is found in persons who consume large quantities of alcohol (a quart or more of whiskey a day) over a prolonged period. Under these conditions severe withdrawal symptoms are observed. The first detailed and well-controlled study of these phenomena was conducted by Isbell and his co-workers (1955).

Ten men volunteered to drink heavily under medical supervision and then to have their drinking abruptly discontinued. It so happened that the subjects were former morphine addicts. It is unlikely that this influenced the results significantly, because a subsequent study by Mendelson and LaDou (1964) using subjects without any history of drug addiction confirmed the main findings. Nutrition (including vitamins) was carefully controlled, thus proving that the withdrawal symptoms were not due merely to nutritional deficiencies.

A picture of typical symptoms after removal of alcohol can be gained from the following description:

> Tony, who drank for 48 days, was still intoxicated, joking and sing-ing 8 hours after his last drink. . . . As his blood alcohol level declined he became extremely tremulous and weak, perspired freely, gagged, retched and vomited. Fourteen hours after discontinuance of alcohol he had to be helped into a chair. . . . Sixteen hours after his last drink . . . he stated he had seen a naked woman and a big yellow spot on the wall. . . . Throughout the first night of abstinence he was unable to sleep, complained of extreme nervousness, perspired profusely, had a marked tremor, diarrhea, and a variety of hallucinations (Isbell et al., 1955, p. 24–25).

On the sixth day, because of Tony's extreme agitation it had been decided that it was too dangerous to continue the experiment, and Tony was sedated so that he could sleep at night and not be agitated during the day. Fourteen days after his last drink Tony appeared normal.

Use of Alcohol in Moderation

Judicious use of alcohol does not lead to alcoholism. As McClelland (1971) says in an article with the intriguing title "The power of positive drinking," a drink or two is a pleasant way to relax with friends and enjoy a feeling of mild exhilaration. There is wide agreement these days that well-modulated drinking is safe from a biochemical chain of events lead-ing to dependence. Alcohol in small quantities is metabolized readily, leaving the cellular environment the same as before. But taking morphine in comparable amounts (that is, enough to produce pleasurable effects) is liable to initiate tissue changes that lead to dependence.

Discussion in detail of possible biochemical and pharmacological mechanisms in alcoholism is beyond the scope of this book. In general, there are two kinds of hypotheses guiding research in this area at the present time. The first suggests that the continuous ingestion of very large quantities of alcohol may cause deviations in the normal metabolism of alcohol, resulting in the formation of compounds capable of producing physical dependence. According to the second kind of hypothesis, sudden abstinence, following extremely heavy and continuous alcohol intake, pro-duces a state of disuse (or "denervation") supersensitivity (Jaffe & Sharp-less, 1968), the phenomenon that was noted earlier in connection with morphine dependence.

Again, it seems clear that a large intake of alcohol, enough to produce frequent and prolonged intoxication is required for alcoholism. Therefore, whatever biochemical (and other) conditions underlie *dependence* on alcohol (in the precise meaning of the term *dependence*), they require this enormous intake. However, once the phenomena of the kind described by Isbell are fully developed, almost certainly there is an underlying physiological push mechanism of the kind previously described for thirst (and postulated for morphine dependence). Data from animal experiments support this idea.

Richter (1957) succeeded in producing dependence in three wild rats by restricting their fluid intake to a 10 percent alcohol solution for a period of about 40 days. At the end of the period of forced-feeding with alcohol, the rats continued to drink large quantities of alcohol, even though plain water was made available to them. One animal drank progressively more alcohol and less plain water, ate less and less, and died 30 days later. The course was one that closely parallels that of some human alcoholics.

In domesticated rats, however, Richter states that, even with more prolonged periods of forced-feeding of alcohol, no such clear signs of dependence were ever observed. It is possible that dependency in the domesticated rat could be demonstrated with still longer periods of exposure to alcohol. But Richter found no such difference between wild and domesticated rats when force-fed for three to six months on diets supplemented with increasingly higher concentrations of morphine sulfate. Wild and domesticated rats showed very similar withdrawal symptoms when the morphine sulfate was removed from the diet. (It will be recalled that other workers reported clear-cut dependence on morphine in domesticated rats.) The available evidence from animals is in line with clinical knowledge that dependence on morphine is much more readily established than is dependence on alcohol. That dependence is much more common in the case of tobacco than alcohol has been commented on recently by Brain (1965).

From research on human alcoholism (Isbell et al., 1955; Mendelson & LaDou, 1964) we know that large quantities of alcohol (for example, a liter or more of whiskey a day) must be drunk over a prolonged period in order to produce severe withdrawal symptoms. It required considerable ingenuity to make animals drink ethanol in sufficient volumes to drive their blood alcohol to intoxicating levels. Recently a few investigators have succeeded in doing this.

Ellis and Pick (1970) gave ethanol (alcohol) by gastric intubation to rhesus monkeys: "Termination of ethanol administration after 10 to 18 days of treatment resulted in the emergence, during the withdrawal periods, of a series of hyperexcitability signs which could be classified into tremulous, spastic and convulsive stages." Declining blood-ethanol concentrations showed correlations with the progressive severity of symptoms;

and it was possible to reverse these symptoms by the administration of ethanol. Subsequently, these investigators obtained similar results with dogs and, in addition, reported that "the administration of various daily doses of ethanol for varying periods of time produced a variety of withdrawal patterns, suggesting that both dose- and time-dependent relationships may be important in the induction of dependence on ethanol" (Ellis & Pick, 1972).

Pieper, Skeen, McClure, and Bourne (1972) put alcohol in the formulas of infant chimpanzees who drank the alcohol and liquid diet mix in their baby bottles at scheduled feeding times. At first the chimpanzees refused to drink the solution if it contained alcohol. However, by commencing with weak solutions and gradually increasing the alcohol concentration, the experimenters contrived to get the animals to drink large quantities of alcohol in concentrations strong enough to produce high blood-alcohol levels.

After 6 to 10 weeks, when alcohol was abruptly removed from the diet, all six chimpanzees showed withdrawal symptoms. Extremely severe symptoms, including convulsions, were observed in three animals, one of whom died after prolonged and repeated convulsions. In the course of these studies, tolerance to ethanol was also observed. Pieper and Skeen (1972) obtained positive results in similar experiments using young rhesus monkeys as subjects. Falk, Samson, and Winger (1972) found that rats maintained on an intermittent food schedule with an available ethanol solution drank to excess. They found that removal of the ethanol produced dependency symptoms including death from convulsions. Previous investigators had failed to produce these effects in rats. The success of Falk and co-workers may be attributed to their ingenious use of the schedule-induced polydipsia (excessive drinking) technique. In relation to the neuropsychological aspect of alcoholism research, there is an interesting development, which will bear watching. Amit, Stern, and Wise (1970) have implicated electrical hypothalamic stimulation in the increased ethanol intake, which they observed in their experiments with rats. A similar (though smaller) effect was observed in M. J. Wayner's laboratory (personal communication, 1973). On the other hand, Martin and Myers (1972) reported negative findings. Current active research on relations between brain stimulation and ethanol intake should resolve these differences.

SUMMARY

There are brain cells (osmoreceptors) whose firing rates increase when the animal needs water. The osmoreceptor is regarded as a key to understanding the neuropsychological mechanisms of internal push, which in interaction with external pull from the environment underlie thirst-related behavior.[4]

It is proposed as a working hypothesis that the neural mechanism underlying cellular dehydration thirst is a prototype for the animal's coping with other inborn needs, and also with the acquired needs associated with drug-taking.

This brings us back to the theme of our archaic brain. When we consider the probable neural correlates of drug addiction, we see the possibility of additional archaic features of the brain: those that make it vulnerable to having its mechanisms for replenishing needed substances perverted to mechanisms of the addictions.

REFERENCES

Amit, Z., Stern, M. H., & Wise, R. A. Alcohol preference in the laboratory rat induced by hypothalamic stimulation. *Psychopharmacologia* (Berl.), 1970, *17*, 367–377.

Andersson, B. Osmoreceptors versus sodium receptors. In A. N. Epstein, H. R. Kissileff, & E. Stellar (Eds.), *The neuropsychology of thirst: New findings and advances in concepts.* Washington, D.C.: Winston, 1973. Pp. 113–116.

Blass, E. M., & Epstein, A. N. A lateral preoptic osmosensitive zone for thirst in the rat. *Journal of Comparative and Physiological Psychology,* 1971, *76*, 378–394.

Brain, L. Drug-dependence. *Nature,* 1965, *208*, 825–827.

Ellis, F. W., & Pick, J. R. Experimentally induced ethanol dependence in rhesus monkeys. *Journal of Pharmacology and Experimental Therapeutics,* 1970, *175*, 88–93.

Ellis, F. W., & Pick, J. R. Ethanol dependence in monkeys and dogs. In J. M. Singh, L. Miller, & H. Lal (Eds.), *Drug addiction: Experimental pharmacology.* Vol. 1. Mount Kisco, N.Y.: Futura, 1972. Pp. 293–300.

Falk, J. L., Samson, H. H., & Winger, G. Behavioral maintenance of high concentrations of blood ethanol and physical dependence in the rat. *Science,* 1972, *177*, 811–813.

Fitzsimons, J. T. Thirst. *Physiological Reviews,* 1972, *52*, 468–561.

Hayward, J. N., & Vincent, J. D. Osmosensitive single neurones in the hypothalamus of unanaesthetized monkeys. *Journal of Physiology,* 1970, *210*, 947–972.

Hebb, D. O. The organization of behavior. New York: Wiley, 1949.

Interim Report of the Commission of Inquiry into the Non-Medical Use of Drugs. Ottawa: Information Canada, 1970.

---

[4] In this chapter, the lateral preoptic area was focused on as the most probable site of central receptors for cellular dehydration thirst. It should be noted, however, that as usual in science, there are alternative points of view. The interested reader may consult Andersson (1973) for a somewhat different view of the problem.

Isbell, H., Fraser, H. F., Wikler, A., Belleville, R. E., & Eisenman, A. J. An experimental study of the etiology of "rum fits" and delirium tremens. *Quarterly Journal of Studies on Alcohol*, 1955, *16*, 1–33.

Jaffe, J. H. Pharmacological approaches to the treatment of compulsive opiate use: Their rationale and current status. In P. Black (Ed.), *Drugs and the brain*. Baltimore, Md.: Johns Hopkins Press, 1969. Pp. 351–362.

Jaffe, J. H., & Sharpless, S. K. Pharmacological denervation supersensitivity in the central nervous system: A theory of physical dependence. *Research Publications, Association for Research in Nervous and Mental Disease*, 1968, *46*, 226–246.

Malmo, R. B., & Mundl, W. J. Osmosensitive neurons in the rat's preoptic area: Medial-lateral comparison. *Journal of Comparative and Physiological Psychology*, in press.

Martin, G. E., & Myers, R. D. Ethanol ingestion in the rat induced by rewarding brain stimulation. *Physiology and Behavior*, 1972, *8*, 1151–1160.

McClelland, D. C. The power of positive drinking. *Psychology Today*, 1971, *4*, 40–79.

Mendelson, J. H., & LaDou, J. Experimentally induced chronic intoxication and withdrawal in alcoholics. Part 2. Psychophysiological findings. *Quarterly Journal of Studies on Alcohol*, Suppl. 2, 1964. Pp. 14–39.

Nicolaïdis, S. Étude d'une réponse de sudation après ingestion d'eau chez le sujet déshydraté. *Comptes Rendus des Séances de l'Académie des Sciences*, 1964, *259*, 4370–4372.

Peck, J. W., & Novin, D. Evidence that osmoreceptors mediating drinking in rabbits are in the lateral preoptic area. *Journal of Comparative and Physiological Psychology*, 1971, *74*, 134–147.

Pieper, W. A., & Skeen, M. J. Induction of physical dependence on ethanol in rhesus monkeys using an oral acceptance technique. *Life Sciences*, 1972, *11*, 989–997.

Pieper, W. A., Skeen, M. J., McClure, H. M., & Bourne, P. G. The chimpanzee as an animal model for investigating alcoholism. *Science*, 1972, *176*, 71–73.

Richter, C. P. Production and control of alcoholic cravings in rats. In H. A. Abramson (Ed.), *Neuropharmacology*. New York: Josiah Macy, Jr. Foundation, 1957. Pp. 39–146.

Skinner, B. F. *Science and human behavior*, New York: Macmillan, 1953.

Spragg, S. D. S. Morphine addiction in chimpanzees. *Comparative Psychology Monographs*, 1940, *15*, (7, Whole No. 79).

Stolerman, I. P., & Kumar, R. Preferences for morphine in rats: Validation of an experimental model of dependence. *Psychopharmacologia (Berlin)*, 1970, *17*, 137–150.

Thompson, T., & Ostlund, W., Jr. Susceptibility to readdiction as a function of the addiction and withdrawal environments. *Journal of Comparative and Physiological Psychology*, 1965, *60*, 388–392.

Valenstein, E. S. Biology of drives: A report of an NRP Work Session. *Neurosciences Research Program Bulletin*, 1968, *6*, 1–111.

Verney, E. B. The antidiuretic hormone and the factors which determine its release. *Proceedings of the Royal Society*, 1947, *B135*, 25–106.

Wayner, M. J., & Kahan, S. A. Central pathways involved during the salt arousal of drinking. *Annals of the New York Academy of Sciences*, 1969, *157*, 701–722.

Weeks, J. R. Experimental narcotic addiction. *Scientific American*, 1964, *210* (3), 46–52.

Weeks, J. R., & Collins, R. J. Patterns of intravenous self-injection by morphine-addicted rats. *Research Publications, Association for Research in Nervous and Mental Disease*, 1968, *46*, 288–298.

Wikler, A. Interaction of physical dependence and classical and operant conditioning in the genesis of relapse. *Research Publications, Association for Research in Nervous and Mental Disease*, 1968, *46*, 280–287.

Wolf, A. V. *Thirst*. Springfield, Ill.: Charles C Thomas, 1958.

Wright, J. W. Deviations in food and water consumption and urinary electrolytes with frequency of measurement in rats. *Psychonomic Science*, 1972, *29*, 32–33.

VII

Epilogue

THE SOLE PRODUCT of brain function is muscular coordination; and the entire output of our thinking machine goes into the motor system. These are statements of Sperry's principle, which is one of the main working hypotheses guiding the writing of this book. As Sperry says, comparative neurology teaches us that from the fishes to ourselves there is only a gradual elaboration of brain structures, with persistence of the fundamental principles of operation, and *always the involvement of the motor system*. In short, we think (and perceive things) with brain "machinery" that was "designed" basically for seeking food and water, fleeing from danger, fighting, and the like.

PREDOMINANCE OF THE MOTOR SYSTEM: EMGs AND THE RETICULAR CORE

Documentation for the Sperry principle is abundant, as we noted many times in pursuing the various topics of this book. The extraordinary usefulness of electromyograms (EMGs) in psychological investigations is itself supportive of the principle. The study of Anne's hysterical deafness (and of hypnotic deafness) was greatly assisted by the recording of EMGs, as were the studies of chronic anxiety. In fact, according to Pitts's biochemical theory of anxiety, excessive muscular contraction is the *sine qua non* of chronic anxiety.

A major part of Chapter III is devoted to descriptions of electromyographic (EMG) gradients, which have been observed in a wide variety of organized activities (such as performing a task, listening to a story, engaging in an interview). EMG gradients appear in certain muscle groups only. Where the gradients appear depends on the situation and on the individual. When tension rises high enough it produces pain. Some individuals who are prone to develop high-amplitude EMG gradients in the forehead muscles, for example, have frequent frontal headaches. The muscles at the back of the neck are another source of frequently recurring painful tension in many people.

These pervasive EMG gradients are considered to be largely a function of the reticular core, which is described in Chapter V. According to our theory, the total brain mechanism for any complexly organized and goal-directed behavior sequence must include facilitation from the firing of neurons in the reticular core. Furthermore, according to our theory, progressively increasing facilitation is required in order to overcome the progressive adaptation ("fatigue") of higher-order neurons in the neocortex and elsewhere in the brain, during the course of the behavior sequence. The EMG gradients appear, it is suggested, because the muscle fibers are much more resistant to adaptation than are central neurons, and so reflect in the EMGs the increasing facilitatory bombardment from the reticular core.

The downstream facilitation from the reticular core is important, in its own right, for the mediation of any behavior sequence, although the question of the role of the muscles per se remains an undecided point. It is the *motor system* (as defined in Chapter III) that is indispensable. The *muscles* themselves *may* be superfluous for thinking, as most people believe. However, clear evidence on this point appears to be lacking. The frequently cited experiment by Smith and his co-workers (Chapter III) fails to prove, as some secondary sources erroneously state, that the person whom they paralyzed with curare could *think* coherently. No valid tests of thinking were administered. Although the subject remained conscious and was able to recall things that happened during the period of paralysis, he did state that he found it difficult to focus his attention. This and other research, which was reviewed, raise serious doubt about concluding, on the basis of present evidence, that normal muscular activity is superfluous for attentiveness.

Circulation of the blood, respiration, and other autonomic nervous system functions (Chapter IV) play a supportive role in relation to activity of the skeletal muscles. Excessive activation of these functions forms the basis of bodily complaints in some patients whom we studied: complaints such as rapid beating of the heart, chest pains, difficulties with breathing, high blood pressure, and the like. Some persons are more prone to distress from such autonomic dysfunctions than they are to pains from excessive muscular tension. The principle of *symptom specificity* is based on these observations.

Distressing bodily symptoms, such as tension headache, have been treated by using feedback techniques (commonly called "biofeedback"). In this appproach to bodily symptoms, attempts have been made to gain control over autonomic functions, something that was considered impossible a decade or so ago. The wise influence of Neal Miller in this fascinating research area has both stimulated a substantial number of experiments and introduced a note of healthy caution. Results of EMG feedback treatment of tension headaches appear especially promising (Chapter IV).

Electromyography (and other related physiological measures) are good indices of the *effort* a person is making in performing a task. In experiments where degree of effort was varied in accordance with graded incentives, Stennett showed that the optimal condition for performance was moderately high incentive, which was associated with a moderate level of muscle tension (that is, moderately steep EMG gradient). With *extremely* high incentive and *extremely* steep EMG gradients, performance suffered. (It is common knowledge that one can "try too hard.") Goodman's experiments with monkeys demonstrated a similar relation between performance and level of neuronal activity recorded from the reticular core. Again, a moderate level was more favorable than levels of neuronal firing that were either too low or too high.

Both of these experimental findings support our hypothesis that beyond a certain level neuronal activation in the reticular core is unfavorable for good performance. Applying this working hypothesis to field observations in disaster situations and on the battlefield, it appears that the reticular core (and related brain structures with facilitation on the motor system) can become so overactivated that they have devastating effects on performance. This is interpreted as still another manifestation of the troubles caused by our archaic brain. There are also troubles on the *sensory* side, and we now review one of them.

ON SENSORY MECHANISMS IN THE BRAIN THAT SIGNAL NEEDS

Chapter VI discusses recent research on osmoreceptors, which are central receptors for detecting cellular dehydration. The discovery of osmoreceptors is exceedingly important for the psychology of thirst because it provides a biologically meaningful *point of origin* from which to work toward a basic understanding of the neural mechanisms underlying thirst and drinking behavior. In the recorded neural activity of osmo-receptors, we have what appears to be an exceedingly valuable clue to a source of *internal push.*

The concept of interaction between internal push and *selective pull,* instigated by external cues, was introduced in the context of brain functions and behavior. This concept of interaction was then extended to a discussion of morphine addiction and alcoholism considered as "acquired needs." This neuropsychological approach proved helpful in eliminating the dualistic distinction between "psychological" and "physical" dependence, and in suggesting some new lines of experimental attack on the problems of drug addiction. These perspectives also served to expose still another archaic feature of our brain, that is, the perversion of our need-signaling systems to the addictions.

ON EMOTIONS

The first point to be noted is that it is impossible to solve *the* problem of emotion, for the reason that the phenomena that psychologists have collected under the heading of "emotions" are too heterogeneous to permit any general solution. The question, "What is emotion?" has produced controversies but few useful concepts.

The most famous controversy was that between William James and Walter B. Cannon. In brief, the former attempted to reduce the *experience* of emotions to *mere feedback* from a fast-beating heart, increased breathing rate, and the other physiological consequences of sympathetic activation (described in Chapter IV). James attributed the sympathetic activation to sheer association of the stimulating situation with past danger. Some of Cannon's objections to James's theory were: (a) sympathetic activation is generalized so that there can be no distinctive physiological patterns from emotion to emotion, (b) autonomic changes are relatively slow so that if the feedback hypothesis were correct, a feeling of fright, for example, would not occur as quickly as experience tells us it does occur (that is, within a half-second), (c) emotional behavior can still occur after surgery that removes the structures for sympathetic activation.

Adrenalin as a Source of Internal "Push": Schachter and Singer Experiment

From Chapter II it will be recalled that secretion of adrenalin (the main neurotransmitter for the sympathetic nervous system) prepares the skeletal muscles for action. In this sense, increased adrenalin in the blood stream may be regarded as a source of internal push (or *arousal*). Schachter and Singer (1962) injected adrenalin into persons, who did indeed feel aroused. However, the state of feeling that they reported after injection depended on whether or not they had received an appropriate explanation of the effects of adrenalin. After the injection and explanation, the person went out to a waiting room where a stooge was engaged in euphoric acts, dancing about, sailing a paper airplane in the air, and so on. The stooge invited the subject to join him in this nonsensical behavior. Persons who were given an appropriate explanation ("You are trembling and your heart is racing") were annoyed by the stooge's antics, and refused the stooge's invitation. On the other hand, misinformed subjects ("You feel numb") did join in and were thoroughly amused by the tomfoolery.

The Schachter-Singer experiment demonstrates the critical importance of the interaction between (a) the physiological arousal caused by the adrenalin injection, and (b) the explanation that was given. This *interaction* determined the subject's feelings in the test situation.

The results of this experiment illustrate the value of looking for interactions between internal *push* (arousal) and external *pull* (social facilitation) factors. The "quick emotion" produced by adrenalin injection also provides a sharp contrast with the long-persisting and intense emotions of chronic anxiety.

Chronic Anxiety

The main problem raised by chronic anxiety is accounting for the persistence of intense internal push. In concrete terms, why do those airmen described in Chapter II fail to "snap out of it" in a few days after being removed to a rest center away from the battle lines? In other words, why do they need such a long period of time in which to recover?

The same problem exists in accounting for the persistence of chronic anxiety in civilian life (incidence: about one person in twenty). In fact, the term "free-floating" anxiety is often applied to the feelings these people have, because there is no obvious connection between their feelings of anxiety and their restful surroundings. Typically, after some months of hard-driving work under difficult circumstances, the person who has been noticing the development of anxiety symptoms (described in Chapter II) finally reaches the point where he has to stop for a period of rest. However, at this point, as in the case of the airman, he cannot relax. His "free-floating" symptoms persist.

According to Pitts's biochemical theory, lactic acid accumulation after excessively long activation of muscle tension is an important factor in anxiety. However, he has found that persons with chronic anxiety metabolize their blood lactic acid as rapidly as normal individuals. Therefore, it seems that we must look elsewhere for an explanation of chronic anxiety.[1] Even without tranquilizing drugs, the person *eventually* recovers. But it takes time. What keeps the tension level so elevated all this time?

Set-Point Hypothesis   The slow time course of the recovery from chronic anxiety suggests that some kind of persisting neural change may be involved. What could it be?

Suppose we examine the chain of events that generally precedes the critical point where a few days of rest are insufficient to remove the disagreeable feelings of strain and the like. There seems to be a factor that is frequently common to both battlefield and civilian chronic-anxiety casualties: a life situation that demands an intense heightening of *effort* over an extended period of time. For the airman it is a series of demanding missions over weeks or months. For the person in civilian life it is a succession of life situations that places intense demands on the individual (Case 3 in Chapter III is an example).

This brings us to the set-point hypothesis. In a common sense way we know that a person working at something will exert effort *up to a certain point*, will put up with so much pressure (or unpleasantness) from others, but beyond a certain point, he will let down, remove himself from unpleasant others and so on. Suppose we regard this point as being analagous to the setting on a thermostat (or a safety valve). When the set-point is reached, the "heat" (so to speak) is turned off. In fact, we actually have a thermostat built into our nervous system. It is designed to keep our internal body temperature at (or very close to) 98.6° Fahrenheit, which is the *set-point* for optimal biological functioning. Now when the person contracts an infectious disease the set-point rises (possibly to combat bacterial invasion) in *fever*. In recovering from the infectious disease, the temperature soon returns to normal.

In order for a set-point mechanism to work, there must be some means for reducing a reaction when it exceeds some critical value. Is there any neurophysiological evidence for a brain mechanism that could do this for muscle contraction? In fact, a mechanism of this kind was discovered twenty-five years ago; but unfortunately, like some other important discoveries, it was insufficiently appreciated at the time.

A Neurophysiological Discovery in Search of a Theory   Jasper (1949) discovered a brain mechanism that damped down excessive muscular activity. Figure 7.1 illustrates one part of Jasper's experiment. The top

---

[1] Ackerman and Sachar (1974) warn against interpreting Pitts's data to mean that peripheral physiological conditions could be causes of anxiety.

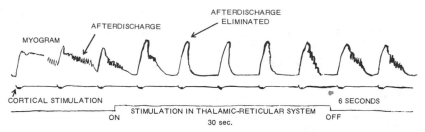

Figure 7.1 *Stimulation in thalamic reticular system of a cat.* Strong electrical stimulation of cat's motor cortex produced response (movement of the hind paw) and motor afterdischarge (muscular activity following response). But when strong electrical stimulation was applied to the motor cortex, and a portion of the thalamic reticular system was stimulated at the same time, the motor afterdischarge was significantly reduced. The cat was lightly anesthetized (see text for explanation). (After H. Jasper, Diffuse projection systems: The integrative action of the thalamic reticular system, *Electroencephalography Clinical Neurophysiology, 1* (1949) 405–420, Fig. 11.)

line in the record is the myogram trace. In the line below this trace, the small dips indicate each point at which Jasper presented brief, very strong, electrical stimulation to the motor area of the cat's neocortex. The cat was lightly anesthetized. There is a place near the top of the brain in the anterior neocortex (that is, the motor cortex) where, upon stimulation, one can elicit movement of the cat's contralateral hind paw. The motor cortex is part of the motor system since it is directly connected with spinal cord motoneurons (by means of the corticospinal tract). The myograph is a mechanical device that registers actual movements of the paw. In this experiment, Jasper's stimulating current was sufficiently strong to produce afterdischarge (that is, movements lasting after the electrical stimulation had ceased). The afterdischarge, it will be noted, was quite pronounced after the first two stimulations.

Now look at the bottom line, which shows when electrical stimulation of another brain area was turned on and off (30 seconds later). Notice that the steady stimulation in the second brain area (thalamic reticular system) had the effect of reducing the *afterdischarge* of the third response (which had been elicited prior to thalamic reticular stimulation), greatly reducing the fourth, and abolishing afterdischarge in the next three responses. After about 25 seconds of thalamic reticular stimulation there was slight return of afterdischarge. Yet the effectiveness of the thalamic reticular stimulation in reducing the *excess* motor reaction was remarkable.

It is important to point out that stimulation of this thalamic reticular area abolished afterdischarge, without affecting the first part of the response. As will be explained presently, the motor reaction prior to the introduction of thalamic stimulation resembles that of anxiety patients to loud sound (see Figure 2.1).

Until the discovery of the reticular systems, the thalamus was regarded mainly as a way station (a relay center) for sensory pathways going toward the cerebral cortex. The thalamic reticular system differs in organizational pattern from the midbrain reticular formation and should not be regarded as merely a simple extension of the midbrain reticular core. However, there are projections from the midbrain reticular core to the thalamic reticular system, as well as the reverse: from thalamic reticular system to the reticular core of the upper midbrain. Furthermore, there are pathways from neocortex to the thalamic-reticular system.

The effect of the thalamic reticular stimulation in reducing after-discharge is an *inhibitory* effect. There is a part of the lower brain-stem reticular core that, when stimulated, has an *inhibitory* effect on muscular activity.

A word of explanation should be given concerning *neural inhibition*, which may seem mysterious to some readers. Actually, neural inhibition is the mirror image of neural excitation. The nerve cell in its resting state has positive ions on the outside and negative ions on the inside, separated by a *semipermeable* membrane, which allows some ions to pass through but not others. According to chemical theories of neural transmission, when an *excitatory* neurotransmitter reaches a critical concentration on the nerve cell, the outer surface of the neuron becomes *negative*. At this point the membrane is depolarized. The spread of depolarization down a fiber (nerve or muscle fiber) was described in Chapters I and III. On the other hand, when an *inhibitory* neurotransmitter reaches a critical concentration on the nerve cell, it *hyper*polarizes the cell body, making it *harder* for the excitatory transmitter to depolarize it.

Figure 7.2 presents a diagram showing how Jasper's neurophysiological mechanism could be extended to provide the kind of set-point control that we have been considering. The downward projection from the thalamic reticular system to the inhibitory portion of the brain-stem reticular system is likely the pathway responsible for the inhibition of after-discharge which Jasper observed. The ascending pathway to the thalamic reticular system from the spinal cord (via the cerebellum) is the pathway that we discussed in Chapter III in relation to Hodes' experiment. In the set-point mechanism that we are considering, this pathway would feed in information about the intensity of muscular contraction. It will be recalled from Chapter III that impulses from muscle and tendon receptors are carried in the spinal columns directly to the cerebellum, which has an input to the reticular core of the brain stem. The transmission would go as follows: muscle receptors to cerebellum, to brain-stem reticular core, up to the thalamic reticular system. If the muscular activity were sufficiently strong, the thalamic reticular neurons would be fired, and their impulses reaching the inhibitory part of the lower brain stem would cause

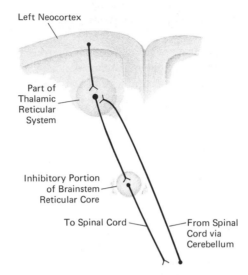

Left Neocortex

Part of
Thalamic
Reticular
System

Inhibitory Portion
of Brainstem
Reticular Core

To Spinal Cord

From Spinal
Cord via
Cerebellum

Figure 7.2   *Diagram illustrating hypothetical neural mechanism for raising set-point for thalamic reticular damping of excessive muscular contractions.*   Upper encircled portion represents the part of the thalamic reticular system where Jasper stimulated. The diagram represents part of a vertical (cross-sectional) view of the brain. This thalamic area lies above the cross-hatched area in Figure 5.3. The location of the thalamus is also shown in Figure 4.1D. The part of the thalamic reticular system that Jasper stimulated is shown as being in the left hemisphere, and the muscle mechanisms are represented as contralaterally placed, on the right side. The diagram illustrating this hypothetical multineuronal mechanism is greatly simplified. In addition to being elaborately multineuronal, the actual neural pathways will undoubtedly turn out to utilize neural networks, and these pathways probably include several other brain structures intercalated between the ones indicated in the diagram.

the inhibitory neurons there to hyperpolarize certain motoneurons in the spinal cord, reducing the level of muscle activity.

So far then, the mechanism essential for checking high-level muscle activity is sketched in. The pathway from the neocortex to the thalamic reticular system is a (hypothetical) source of inhibitory impulses, which would effectively *raise* the set-point. This would be accomplished by its hyperpolarizing some of the neurons in the thalamic reticular system so that the ascending excitatory impulses would have to be increased in strength in order to discharge them, which would allow a higher-than-normal level of muscle activity.

Such a system as this would work well (along with augmentation of supportive autonomic functions) in providing for extra muscular exertion (extra effort) to meet emergencies; and by the return of the set-point to normal afterwards, the motor system would have a built-in protection against excessive strain. (For a parallel to this in autonomic functions, see the description in Chapter IV of the carotid sinus mechanism and the overriding influence of the cortical-hypothalamic-midbrain mechanism.)

If, however, extremely demanding life situations are prolonged over weeks and months, it seems the set-point *sticks* at the higher (above normal) level even when the individual is removed to a quiet environment.

With reference to the diagram in Figure 7.2, this could mean that the *inhibitory* input to the thalamic reticular system would continue to operate (a state of affairs that is now inappropriate to the nondemanding environmental situation). Possibly long continued transmission through these pathways strengthens certain synaptic connections (akin to what happens in conditioning and learning). This kind of change could be a relatively persistent one, lasting for some months. Eventually, however, in the absence of strong environmental demands, the synaptic connections (through structural or biochemical change) would gradually weaken, somewhat like the extinction of a conditioned response.

This then would be a neural mechanism that could account for the *persistence* of anxiety and the accompanying increase in muscular activity. Recall that the anxiety patient typically reacts to *ordinary* life situations as if they were *emergencies* (Chapter II). Furthermore, if the reader will look again at Figure 2.1, it will be apparent that our EMG data bear significant similarity to the afterdischarge picture in Figure 7.1. Note again that it was the *after*response period that discriminated between anxiety patients and controls, with the former showing significantly *more* after-response than the latter (with no significant difference between the two groups in amplitude of the initial reaction to the stimulus).

Parts of this neural model are admittedly speculative and simplified. For example, the pathway from thalamus to brain stem in Figure 7.2 is probably less direct, involving other structures. However, the neurophysiological findings from Jasper's experiment in the context of twenty-five years of research on the reticular systems encourage the resumption of Jasper's promising neurophysiological approach to motor inhibition. In this further work, the present neural model should be useful in suggesting new experiments.

For our discussion of emotions, this neural model is useful in clarifying the *chronic*[2] nature of pathological anxiety (pathological because of

---

[2] The symptoms of chronic anxiety may persist over months or longer. However, they usually do disappear eventually after some months (especially if treated). Therefore, the term "chronic" is relative. Compared with a brief emotion such as fear, it is indeed chronic. One may speculate about the final outcome in the case of a person whose "set-point" remains elevated for a much longer period (that is, for years instead of months). It seems possible that such persons might fall victim to what Selye (1970) has called "diseases of adaptation," which include ulcers, and cardiovascular and kidney diseases.

its inappropriateness and for its source of extremely unpleasant feelings that the anxiety patient experiences over a long period of time). In sharp contrast with chronic anxiety, *fear* is quickly elicited and usually has a short time course.

Fear

An adult person (or chimpanzee) seeing a snake normally retreats, showing signs that an observer would interpret as those of fear. This fear of snakes is not learned; neither are fears instigated by such things as darkness in a strange place. Human adults (but not very young children) react with fear (or horror) to distorted and damaged human bodies. The age factor is important in fear reactions. Children rarely show fear in darkness before the age of three, but show it frequently thereafter. Human infants show no fear of strangers until they are six months old.

These fears represent something more than anticipation of danger (because in many instances no danger is involved). In general, fear seems to be caused by some perceptual incongruity (or discrepancy), something that intrudes itself into well-developed perceptual sequences, breaking the perceptual continuity and causing visible disruption of an ongoing behavior sequence.[3] This behavioral disruption may take the form of strong facilitation on the motor system (such as screaming and panic-stricken flight in chimpanzees on seeing a "death mask").

From this discussion it is clear that fear and chronic anxiety are distinctly different; although both cause disruption of behavior sequences, they present vastly different problems.

There is also an enormous difference between long-enduring resentment and a brief bout of anger. As we noted in Chapter IV, the former can be a strong contributing factor in Raynaud's disease (characterized by painful constriction of the peripheral blood vessels). Transient bouts of anger on the other hand have no such long-term consequences.

It is thus apparent that preoccupation with the question, "What is emotion?" is useless. What we should be asking is "What can we learn about this particular behavior and its physiological accompaniments?" We can regard the term *emotion* as denotative: that is, a handy shorthand notation that the behavior falls into a *category* designated as "emotional." In other words, for scientific analysis, we are required to formulate specific questions. We have dealt with a few specific questions in the area of the

[3] D. O. Hebb (1966) is responsible for marshaling the evidence supporting many of my statements about fear. Hebb also calls attention to other irrational and apparently nonlearned fears we have, such as those that cause us to react (with fear and distrust) against the strange (including people who are different from ourselves in some way).

emotions. Of course, there are many other questions (many other problems), but space does not permit discussion of them in this book.

One further point: sometimes emotions are discussed as though they are the *exceptions* to "normal" smooth-running emotion-free behavior sequences. However, the obvious fallacy in this notion (besides the fact that emotions can have an organizing effect) was discussed in Chapter III in connection with Nauta's principle, and the manifestations of our *archaic brain*.

Nauta's principle, it will be recalled, is illustrated by the roads on roads example. In its evolution, the brain has progressed in a rather stupid manner. Like the building of a new highway by paving over only half an old dirt road, our brain's advances are also closely associated with and at times dominated by structures that may be identified (as having changed very little) through the whole mammalian series. Now let us briefly review some manifestations of our archaic brain, which we have discussed earlier.

OUR ARCHAIC BRAIN

Archaic means "belonging to or having the characteristics of an *earlier, more primitive time.*" In this book, archaic is applied to the human brain: *the whole brain* (not just a part of the brain, such as the limbic system or the reticular system).

In primitive times, the human, like other animals, had to meet certain emergency situations (attack by a predator, attacking another animal for food, fleeing, and so on). Physiological mechanisms that are well suited to meeting emergencies have been understood since W. B. Cannon's classical writings. However, in modern times, in adjusting to life situations structured by "civilization," these same mechanisms are sometimes activated continuously over long periods of time. In other words, physiological mechanisms that were designed for *short-term* use are now constantly used for *long-term* social strivings.

In this book, we have discussed the consequences of the strains thus produced by these inappropriate physiological activations: chronic anxiety, tension headaches, high blood pressure (hypertension), Raynaud's disease, and other symptoms related to the heart and circulation of blood. In examining all of these disorders, it was evident that overly strong facilitation on the *motor system* was a common factor.

As previously noted, the human brain is archaic in another respect: where the neurophysiological function under scrutiny is *sensory*. Reference is made again to the topic of brain receptors for detecting cellular dehydration (Chapter VI).

If, as seems likely, receptor cells like these "give themselves over to" morphine addiction or alcoholism, then they, too, are plainly part of an archaic mechanism. It is interesting to note that one definition of *addicted* is "given up, or over to."

A third way in which our brains are archaic was discussed in Chapter V, and it was also mentioned earlier in this chapter. Again, the physiological mechanisms for emergency are implicated, but in a different way than in the case of chronic anxiety, tension headaches, and so on. We noted how, under modern battlefield conditions, activation of *flight* results in the so-called panic run (Chapter V). Too, the *freezing* response, useful to an animal hiding from a predator, was shown to be completely maladaptive in certain battle situations. A related paralyzing inhibition of coordinated behavior is observed in disaster situations (Chapter V). These fatal inadequacies of primitive neurophysiological response mechanisms in man-made situations are plainly archaic.

Finally, there is an important point that was mentioned in the preceding section on *fear*. We react with fear to strange perceptions. In short, many of our fears are irrational. Inherent distrust of the strange and different, it may be noted, could prevent a valuable mutation in human kind from making extraordinarily important contributions. For example, a greatly enlarged cranium to accommodate an oversized brain in a mutant would appear grotesque; and this grotesque appearance might easily make it impossible for the superintelligent mutant to gain the confidence of other persons.

MacLean's Conception of the "Triune Brain"

Paul MacLean also believes that the human brain is archaic. MacLean divides the human brain into three main parts, which he places in a hierarchical schema: (a) reptilian brain, (b) paleomammalian brain (limbic system), and (c) neomammalian brain (neocortex).

In our review of the central nervous system, the reticular core and midbrain correspond most closely to the reptilian brain, which is the most primitive one, in MacLean's hierarchy. Reptiles depend almost entirely on subcortical structures. In contrast to mammals there is only a rudimentary cortex. There is basic agreement between the primary role of these primitive midbrain (and other) structures in MacLean's triune and our emphasis on the critical role of the midbrain and the motor system in the mediation of behavior (see Chapter III).

The paleomammalian counterpart of the human brain corresponds to the limbic system, which was given this name by MacLean in 1952. The limbic system was discussed in Chapter III in relation to monkey vocalizations (see Figure 3.16 and explanatory text). In addition to the limbic cortex, MacLean includes some parts of the brain stem with which the limbic cortex has primary connections. MacLean believes that the primitive limbic cortex gives the lower mammal improved sensing of internal and external changes. The osmoreceptors, which were discussed in Chapter VI, are examples of limbic sensors of internal change related to thirst. Warning calls in monkeys, which can be reproduced by electrical stimulation of certain limbic structures in the monkeys' brains, are examples of limbic system activation by external changes in the environment.

The neomammalian brain in the neocortex culminates in man to mediate language and complex nonlanguage functions, such as composing music and painting pictures. The unique role of the human neocortex in speech (discussed in Chapter III) seems representative of MacLean's view of the neomammalian brain as the least archaic of the triune.

MacLean's conception of a triune brain is in harmony with the conception of an archaic brain. He believes, for example, that overcompulsiveness is a vestige of reptilian stereotyped behavior; and he has discussed the inevitable intrusion of feelings, mediated by the limbic system, in attempts at objective thinking in science (MacLean, 1970). MacLean thus recognizes the handicaps that are an inevitable outcome of the way the human brain has evolved.

MacLean believes that Freud had the right idea about the archaic nature of our unconscious (unreportable) motivations, but that Freud actually underestimated their importance in the control of behavior (that Freud "drew the id too small").

There is obviously a large measure of agreement between MacLean's formulations and mine. Although different lines of evidence have been offered in each case, they lead to the same kind of conclusion.

My emphasis on the importance of the motor system seems more strongly stated than in MacLean's writings. For example, I am impressed that the projections from the limbic structures diagrammed in Figure 3.16 stop at the midbrain, and thus have no direct facilitation on the skeletal motor system. For this reason, I am perhaps more inclined than MacLean to stress the merging of the limbic system with the midbrain.

EVOLUTION AND GENETICS

The human brain is, of course, a product of the evolutionary process. Up to now it has been good enough for survival. But there is evidence to suggest that the evolutionary process has produced a brain with archaic features. Actually, this should not come as too great a surprise, considering that natural selection is for *mere survival*.

A variation that appears suddenly in a species and then is transmitted to offspring is a *mutation*. Mutations involve an alteration in the structure of a chromosome (the small body taking part in the cell division in the fertilized ovum, which carries genes, the determiners of hereditary traits).

Mutations were obviously responsible for evolutionary advances in plants and animals over the past billion years. Mutations may be induced by exposing plants and animals to mutagens (radiation or certain chemicals).

Mutations are induced (by radiating the seeds) in plants to improve them in various ways (Sigurbjörnsson, 1971). Mutant rice, which has been developed in Japan, reaches maturity about two months earlier and has seeds with more protein than the older type of rice. Wheat was improved in Italy by mutation. The older variety was satisfactory when grown in unfertilized soil, but in fertilized soil it bent to the ground during wind and rain. The mutant wheat is shorter and has stronger stalks and so remains standing upright under all weather conditions. In the United States, direct mutation breeding in the peppermint plant succeeded (where other methods had failed) in producing a plant that was resistant to a wilt disease, which was threatening the billion-dollar-a-year peppermint oil industry.

There are many other applications of induced mutations in plant breeding; and future use of this technique seems exceedingly promising.

It was the American geneticist and Nobel Prize winner H. J. Muller who discovered that mutations are increased following irradiation of the fruit fly *Drosophila* with X-rays. The discovery that the same technique can be used to produce mutations in plants was made by another American worker, L. J. Stadler. There were some initial difficulties with the method as applied by plant breeders; but, as previously mentioned, the future of mutant plants looks promising for agriculture.

With regard to research with animals, geneticists have found that it is possible to identify the genetic components of behavior by working with mutations in fruit flies. Benzer (1973) states that his:

> objectives are to discern the genetic component of a behavior, to identify it with a particular gene and then to determine the actual site at which the gene influences behavior and learn how it does so. . . . Although the fly's nervous system is very different from the human system, both consist of neurons and synapses and utilize transmitter molecules, and the development of both is dictated by genes. . . . Its nervous system is a miracle of microminiaturization, and some of its independently evolved behavior patterns are not unlike our own (p. 24).

NEUROPSYCHOLOGY IN RELATION TO "GENETIC ENGINEERING"

We must see the possibilities in these developments in genetics for advancing our own evolution. (The term one hears nowadays is *genetic engineering.*) Some people fear that the application of genetic knowledge could be premature (or contrived to give some social groups advantages over others). Marshall W. Nirenberg, the biochemist whose brilliant work was the first giant stride toward cracking the genetic code, has warned that we will be able to manipulate our genes before we are sufficiently knowledgeable about the consequences of such manipulations.

We should regard these developments as challenges to neuropsychology—which is obviously one of the key sciences with responsibility for discovering critical relations between genes and behavior. Of course, it will be many years (possibly centuries) before there can be any wise application of mutagens to people (if indeed it will ever occur). Many (perhaps most) people believe that tampering with genes may threaten our future. At the same time, we must see that the knowledge from behavioral genetics will be valuable in any event. Such knowledge could well prevent premature use of mutagens. Clearly, a most important requirement for steering a wise course through *these* dangerous waters is a profound knowledge of brain function in relation to behavior.

SCIENCE FICTION AND PSYCHOLOGY

We are living in an age to appreciate the old saying that today's science fiction is tomorrow's science. Before me as I write are two pictures. One picture is of Edwin E. Aldrin, Jr., placing a lunar seismometer on the lunar surface, with jet black space in place of sky. This picture was taken by Neil A. Armstrong on July 20, 1969. The other picture was taken by the Apollo 11 astronauts on their way to the moon. It shows our earth as a small multicolored sphere in black space. Is it not easy to imagine an artist's version of these pictures as illustrations in a science fiction book of the 1950s?

The most famous science fiction book about psychology is B. F. Skinner's *Walden Two*. It has sold about a million copies since its publication in 1948.

Skinner's great contribution to psychology is his formulation of *operant conditioning*. He is most famous for his invention of the device that is used to study operant conditioning: called the Skinner box (by everyone except Skinner himself). One example of its use is Weeks's experiment with morphine-dependent rats (Chapter VI). The fact that a rat will press a lever to inject himself with morphine demonstrates the reward value of morphine. The Skinner box was also used by Olds and Milner in their proof that brain stimulation can be rewarding (Chapter IV). The rat's learning to press the lever for reward is operant learning (or conditioning). Hundreds of psychologists have used the device for myriad research problems. However, Skinner avoids the problems of explaining how the brain works and concentrates upon finding out how best to modify and control behavior through *reinforcement* (rewards).

Walden Two is a utopian experimental community where poverty and selfish competitiveness are eliminated, and where the people share the joys of working and living. Every person in this joyful community has a light share of irksome chores, as well as shared care of the children; but each person has time to be creative. Near the end of this book, it is revealed that this utopian existence is brought about through techniques of reinforcement (reward) and learning.

While the science fiction of *Walden Two* comes nowhere near the kind of fruition that journeys to the moon represent (in realizing Jules Verne's dreams of space travel), still the *Walden Two* concept is now actually being tested in communes across the United States.

Therefore, one should not *prejudge* the potential effectiveness of operant learning techniques in reaching Skinner's goals, which without any doubt *are* utopian. Skinner is sure they will work if they are applied correctly. I am much less optimistic, because I believe that in order to ascend to the utopia of *Walden Two* (in order to apply Skinner's *complete plan*) we need better brains than any now in existence. In short, I believe that Skinner fails to perceive just how archaic our brains are. Therefore, I suggest that other authors should write companion novels as exercises in suggesting how the neurosciences could help to produce a better brain!

As a first step, suppose we sketch out a neuropsychological science fiction plot, basing it on some facts that were discussed earlier in the book.

In Chapter III it was explained that monkey vocalization appears to be chiefly a product of the limbic system, whereas human speech is neocortically mediated. Moreover, from what is known about the circuitry of the human brain it seems possible for human speech (and verbalized thought) to occur *at times* without involving the limbic system. It was explained that this partial independence of brain mechanisms for speech from limbic system structures represents an enormous advance over the monkeys, whose vocalizations seem to be exclusively devoted to functions mediated by the limbic system: aggressive attack, warning against predators, fleeing from them, and the like, in addition to activities promoting survival of the individual (drinking and eating), and of the species (mating).

The neuroscientist in our science fiction story devotes his research to altering the genetic determiners for that part of the monkey's motor system that controls the muscles essential for phonation: those of breathing, the small muscles attached to laryngeal cartilages, which control the closing of the vocal folds so that they can be thrown into vibration, the muscles of the tongue, lips, jaws, and so on. The aim would be to provide a motor system for complex phonation, with extensive neocortical connections but with radically reduced limbic connections. In short, the neuroscientist's goal is to use mutagens in order to create a monkey with a brain mechanism for vocalization that is more like our own, with rich connections between the entire apparatus for speech (including its neocortical motor control) and association areas in the neocortex. Now when the monkey's motor cortex is stimulated, he would vocalize just as a person does when stimulated in the corresponding area (Broca's area).

The next development in the plot has the monkey using his vocalization (now largely freed from limbic system domination) to learn to speak, under the tutelage of a linguist.

As the story continues, a breed of monkeys with capacity for speech[4] is developed. Speech training is commenced when the monkeys are very young, and the brighter ones learn to carry on conversations with people. There are some difficulties in teaching the animals to speak properly, because their motor mechanism for speech is relatively limited. However, despite these difficulties, it is possible for psychologists to study their capacities for thinking and for verbalizing their thoughts. The psychologists report that although the monkeys' capacities for thinking are rather limited, the thinking of the mutant monkeys seems more dispassionate (and more compassionate) than the thinking of most humans. The precise words from one of the reports was, "The subject seems to possess the capacity for wholly dispassionate cognition, and at the same time to be deeply considerate of the welfare and wishes of others. Selfish (ego-centered) motivation seems to be absent."

These findings were most puzzling at first. However, eventually the neuroscientists came to recognize that in certain respects these mutant monkeys possessed brains that were less archaic than their own. On this whimsical note we end the sketch for a science fiction story.[5]

This kind of excursion into science fiction can, I believe, be a useful exercise for neuroscientists. I believe that it is heuristic to ask what is wrong with the human brain. Raising questions in this vein could lead us into some new approaches to research on brain function and to a deeper understanding of important relations between brain and behavior.

Neuropsychology is a natural extension of the biological sciences. As psychologists we must see this; and I believe we must make the effort to learn as much as we can about how the brain works. The wonders of the

[4] Psychologists have had some limited success teaching language to chimpanzees (see for example Premack and Premack, 1972). There is also some evidence that electrical stimulation of the chimpanzee neocortex can produce vocalization (Dusser de Barenne, Garol, & McCulloch, 1941; Hines, 1940). Further evidence supporting the absence of neocortical participation in monkeys' vocalizations has just been published. Sutton, Larson, and Lindeman (1974) compared neocortical and limbic lesion effects on monkeys' phonations, and concluded that "control over learned, discriminative phonation in monkeys is not mediated by neocortical regions homologous to human 'speech' areas" (p. 61).

[5] For an entertaining science fiction novel about successive forms of human beings over the next two thousand million years see Stapledon (1930).

human brain are abundantly apparent. Its defects (like our own faults) are harder to see. But as psychologists, we should realize that knowing about our limitations is the key to mature understanding of ourselves; and in the final analysis, our limitations are the limitations of our brains.

REFERENCES

Ackerman, S. H., & Sachar, E. J. The lactate theory of anxiety: A review and reevaluation. *Psychosomatic Medicine*, 1974, *36*, 69–81.

Benzer, S. Genetic dissection of behavior. *Scientific American*, 1973, *229*(6), 24–37.

Dusser de Barenne, J. G., Garol, H. W., & McCulloch, W. S. The "motor" cortex of the chimpanzee. *Journal of Neurophysiology*, 1941, *4*, 287–303.

Hebb, D. O. *A textbook of psychology* (2d ed.). Philadelphia: Saunders, 1966.

Hines, M. Movements elicited from precentral gyrus of adult chimpanzees by stimulation with sine wave currents. *Journal of Neurophysiology*, 1940, *3*, 442–466.

Jasper, H. Diffuse projection systems: The integrative action of the thalamic reticular system. *Electroencephalography and Clinical Neurophysiology*, 1949, *1*, 405–420.

MacLean, P. D. The triune brain, emotion, and scientific bias. In F. O. Schmitt (Ed.), *The neurosciences. Second study program.* New York: Rockefeller University Press, 1970. Pp. 336–349.

Premack, A. J., & Premack, D. Teaching language to an ape. *Scientific American*, 1972, *227*(4), 92–99.

Schachter, S., & Singer, J. E. Cognitive, social, and physiological determinants of emotional state. *Psychological Review*, 1962, 69, 379–399.

Selye, H. Stress: It's a G.A.S. In A. W. Pressey & J. P. Zubek (Eds.), *Readings in general psychology: Canadian contributions.* Toronto: McClelland & Stewart, 1970. Pp. 382–384.

Sigurbjörnsson, B. Induced mutations in plants. *Scientific American*, 1971, *224* (1), 86–95.

Skinner, B. F. *Walden Two.* New York: Macmillan, 1948.

Stapledon, O. *Last and first men.* Harmondsworth, England: Penguin, 1930.

Sutton, D., Larson, C., & Lindeman, R. C. Neocortical and limbic lesion effects on primate phonation. *Brain Research*, 1974, *71*, 61–75.

AUTHOR INDEX

SUBJECT INDEX

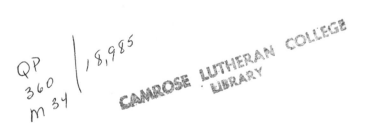